THE
HIGH VITALITY
COOKBOOK

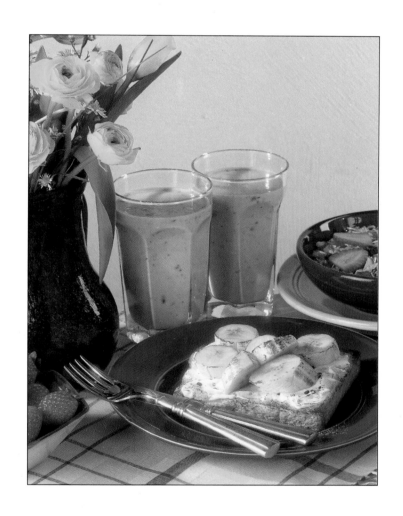

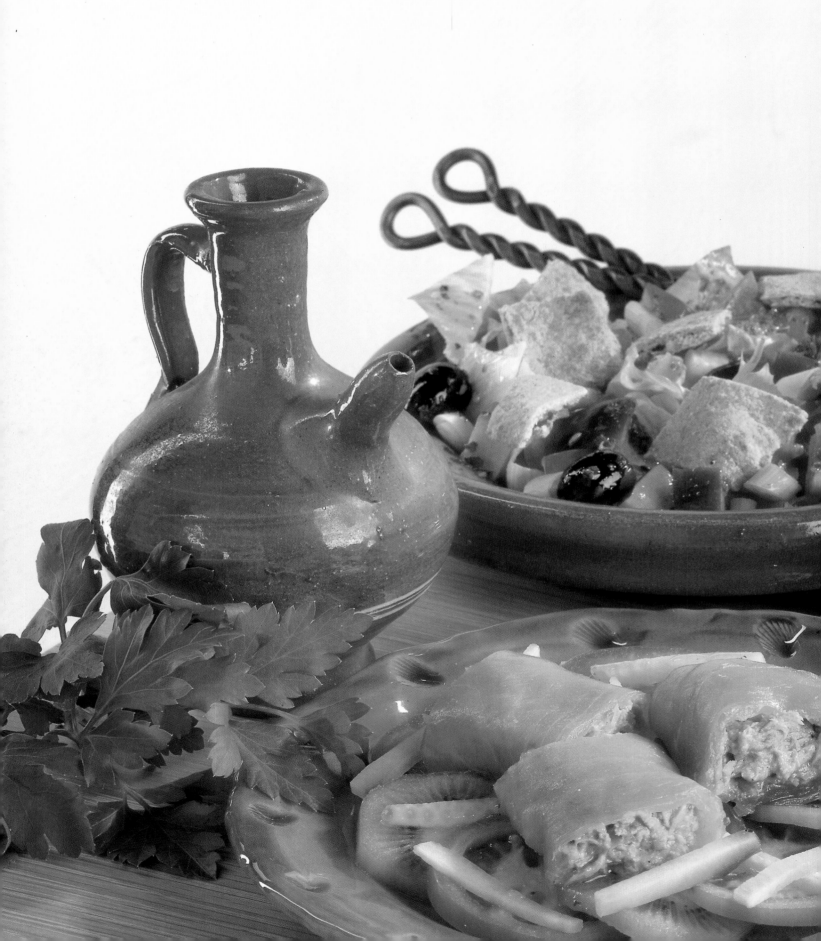

THE HIGH VITALITY COOKBOOK

OVER 70 FABULOUS RECIPES TO IMPROVE HEALTH, ENERGY AND FITNESS

MAGGIE PANNELL

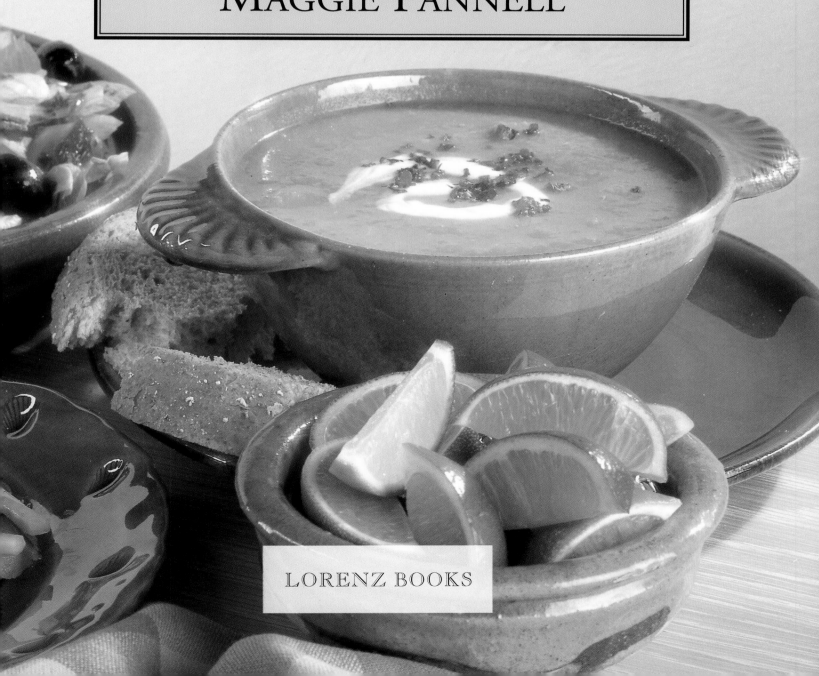

LORENZ BOOKS

This edition published by Lorenz Books
27 West 20th Street, New York, NY 10011

LORENZ BOOKS are available for bulk purchase for sales promotion
and for premium use. For details, write or call the sales director,
Lorenz Books, 27 West 20th Street, New York, NY 10011;
(800) 354-9657

Lorenz Books is an imprint of Anness Publishing Inc.

ISBN 1-85967-884-X

Publisher: Joanna Lorenz
Senior Cookery Editor: Linda Fraser
Cookery Editor: Maggie Mayhew
Designer: Siân Keogh
Photography: Karl Adamson
Food for Photography: Katherine Hawkins
Stylist: Marion McLornan
Illustrator: Madeleine David

Previously published as part of the *Creative Cooking Library*

Printed and bound in Singapore by Star Standard Industries Pte. Ltd.

© Anness Publishing Limited, 1996, 1999

1 3 5 7 9 10 8 6 4 2

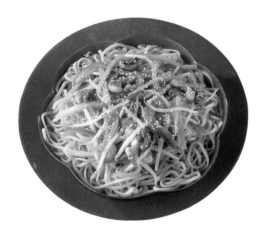

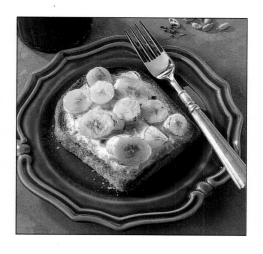
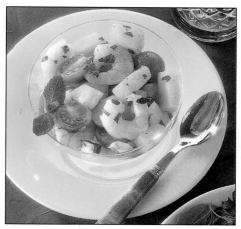
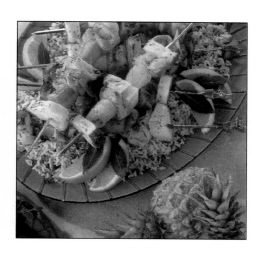

CONTENTS

INTRODUCTION

Do you often feel tired and sluggish? Have you lost that get-up-and-go feeling? How often have you wished you could pack more into your day if only you had the energy? Life is frequently physically and mentally demanding, but it can also be a lot of fun and very rewarding. Naturally, there will always be difficult times and stressful situations that can leave you feeling drained, weary and lethargic, but the good news is that you can have control over how active and alert you feel. Simply by putting the right fuel into your body, you will be able to cope much better with whatever life throws at you. Eat for vitality and you'll discover renewed zest for life, lots more stamina and a more positive outlook.

HOW TO ACHIEVE HIGH ENERGY

It is essential to choose the right balance of foods. Today we are overwhelmed in the supermarket: the shelves are crammed with all kinds of exciting foreign foods, convenience foods and new products. The choice is so enormous that shopping can be quite bewildering.

Also, a great many foods just look so appealing that it's all too easy to be tempted by the photograph on the package and make compulsive purchases rather than make sensible selections based on a sound and informed knowledge of nutrition.

Fortunately, despite some of the unhealthy temptations, there is also a fabulous selection of fresh convenience foods on offer, such as ready-to-use packs of salads and vegetables for stir-frying, which make preparing fresh and wholesome meals quick and easy. Look for healthy eating symbols, such as "high fiber" or "low fat" on food products, although it is wise to read the nutrition panel too, as such claims can often mask other factors, such as a high sugar content.

All food provides nutrients and energy, which is measured in calories. In Western society, there is little likelihood of consuming too few calories (except in cases of eating disorders, such as anorexia nervosa) but there is a real risk of coming up short on essential nutrients, or at least of not getting the best from the food we eat.

This is because certain foods provide much better nutrient value than others. Foods which are lacking in good nutrient value are often said to provide "empty" calories because they contribute little else other than calories, and can therefore be regarded as unnecessary foods (see Foods to Avoid, page 7).

For optimum nutritional and vitality value, choose a fresh wholefood diet containing a wide variety of different foods. This will ensure a good intake of nutrients, particularly the vitamins and minerals essential for helping to generate a good, steady release of energy.

THE ESSENTIAL ENERGIZERS

Although it's very easy to recommend following a balanced diet, in reality diets and eating habits are frequently far from ideal. We rush from appointment to appointment, eat on the run, miss meals, dine out in restaurants or fast-food outlets and seldom stop to think about what we really should be eating. Also, because every individual is different, needs vary, so it is worth considering more closely which nutrients are particularly important in combating fatigue.

The mineral iron is essential for the formation of red blood cells and therefore the oxygen-carrying capacity of the blood. Anemia due to iron deficiency is a common problem in rapidly growing teenagers, women with heavy periods, pregnant women (due to the extra requirement needed

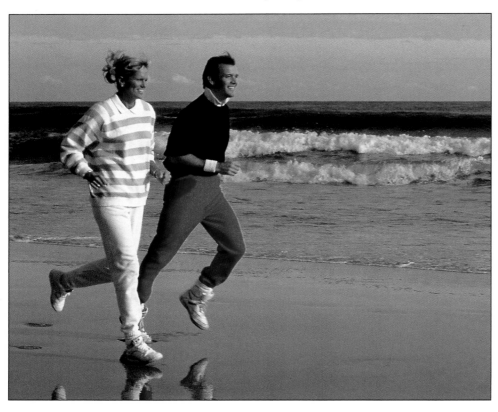

Left: Combine eating a balanced diet with regular exercise.

for a growing baby) and vegetarians who cut out meat without including other good vegetarian sources of iron. Fish helps provide iron.

Zinc deficiency can also contribute to fatigue, and because red meat is the main source from which it is readily absorbed, vegetarians can be at risk if they do not include other sources, like whole-grain cereals, dried fruit, corn on the cob and sesame seeds.

The B-group vitamins are crucial for their role in helping to release energy from food. Vitamin B12 also helps protect against anemia. B-group vitamins are sensitive to heat and are water-soluble, so nutrient-friendly cooking methods should be followed (see Cooking for Vitality, page 9).

Vitamin C helps the body absorb iron from vegetable sources. So, for example, drinking fresh orange or tomato juice with a vegetarian meal will increase the uptake of iron. All fruit and vegetables are sources of vitamin C. Like the B-group vitamins, vitamin C is also unstable and is easily destroyed, so buy fresh and cook quickly or not at all.

Vitamin E also improves the oxygen-carrying capacity of the blood and helps to increase stamina. Good sources of this vitamin include vegetable oils, wheat-germ, eggs, whole wheat bread and nuts.

The key to maximum energy is keeping the blood-sugar level constant. The best foods for doing this are complex, unrefined carbohydrates – whole-grain cereals, dried beans, starchy fruit and vegetables – because they are digested more slowly and release a steady stream of sugar into the blood. These foods are also a good source of dietary fiber, which is essential for a healthy digestive system.

It is important to eat regular meals and not to skip breakfast. The body needs fuel in the morning after its long overnight break. It is also true that those who fail to eat something sustaining for breakfast are much more

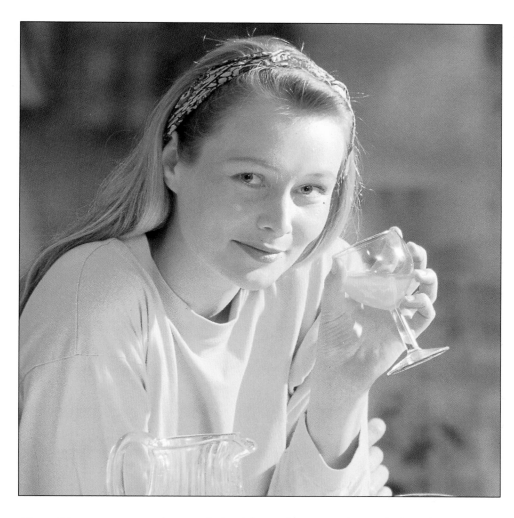

Above: It's important to make time for breakfast and to eat regular meals throughout the day.

likely to snack on whatever is quickest and closest to hand mid-morning, which is unlikely to be a good nutritional choice.

FOODS TO AVOID

The aim should be to cut down on saturated fats, refined carbohydrates and highly processed foods, since these tend to be high in the fats and sugars that pile on unnecessary calories and sap your energy. The list includes most cakes, sweets, chocolates, cookies, fried foods, rich, creamy sauces and pastries. Sugary carbohydrates may give an instant lift, as they are digested quickly and release sugar rapidly into the bloodstream, but the body compensates by releasing a surge of insulin, which pulls the blood-sugar level down low

again, resulting in a sudden drop of energy. Such fluctuations cause tiredness rather than a steady prolonged feeling of well-being. Stimulants, like coffee, tea and alcohol have a similar effect. The caffeine and theobromines in coffee and tea give you a temporary lift, because like alcohol, they cause a rapid release of sugar into the bloodstream, but the effect is short-lived.

These stimulants are also diuretics, so many of the water-soluble vitamins B and C are lost. The tannin in tea inhibits the absorption of iron, and too much caffeine causes insomnia.

Alcohol also depletes stores of vitamins B and C which are needed to detoxify the body. Alcohol and cigarettes both impair the absorption of B vitamins and increase the need for vitamin C.

INGREDIENTS FOR VITALITY

VITALITY DRINKS
Good choices for vitality drinks are decaffeinated coffee, herbal teas or weak Ceylon and China teas, mineral water and fresh fruit juices.

FOODS FOR VITALITY
Whole-grain Cereals: A good source of vegetable protein, iron, B vitamins and vitamin E, whole-grain cereals (brown rice, whole wheat bread and pasta, oats, millet, buckwheat, pearl barley and bulgur) provide much more fiber than refined cereals. Eat plenty of bread, including the many different international varieties, such as Indian nan bread and chapatis, Italian ciabatta (made with olive oil), or Scandinavian and German rye breads. Aim to have about six slices of bread a day – without butter.

Dried Beans: These are good sources of protein, starch carbohydrates, fiber, B vitamins and minerals. If you haven't got time to soak dried beans, canned varieties are just as good. Add them to soups, stews and salads, and experiment with dishes based on beans, lentils and tofu (soy bean curd).

Fruit and Vegetables: Vitamin C is found almost exclusively in fruit and vegetables, and because this vitamin cannot be stored by the body, levels need to be refilled continually. Green

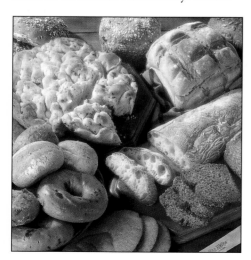

Above: Include a variety of breads, such as ciabatta and German rye bread.

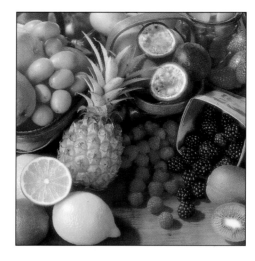

Above: A variety of fresh fruit is important for maintaining vitamin C levels.

vegetables, red bell peppers, citrus fruits, tomatoes, strawberries, kiwi fruit, cranberries and black currants are particularly good sources.

Beta-carotene (which the body converts to vitamin A) and vitamin E are also present in many fruits and vegetables. Several green vegetables, such as broccoli, Brussels sprouts, cabbage, kale and spinach, are excellent sources of beta-carotene as is brightly colored yellow, red and orange produce, such as carrots, apricots, mangoes, peaches and melon. Some good sources of vitamin E include blackberries, asparagus, avocados, broccoli, sweet potatoes, spinach, tomatoes, parsley and watercress.

Fruit and vegetables are also extremely rich in fiber, particularly when eaten with the skin on. Aim to eat at least five portions of fresh fruit and vegetables a day. Use frozen produce when fresh is not available – it is perfectly acceptable from a nutritional point of view.

Dried Fruits: These are an excellent source of minerals, particularly iron, calcium and potassium. Eat raw or cooked for a healthy snack.

Fish: All fish is rich in protein, B vitamins and minerals. White fish is very low in fat. Oily fish, such as sardines, mackerel, herring, tuna, trout

and salmon, also provide vitamins A and D and Omega 3 fatty acids, which are believed to be beneficial in helping to prevent coronary heart disease.

Eggs: Virtually a complete food, eggs provide protein, iron, zinc and vitamins A, B-group and E. However, eggs are not recommended for a low-cholesterol diet. As the yolks are the culprits, egg whites can be substituted, or replace some of the whole eggs.

Poultry: A good source of quality protein, B vitamins and some iron, poultry is also low in fat, particularly if the skin is removed.

Meat and Game: Although the general health advice is to moderate your intake of red meat, thus reducing the amount of saturated fat in your diet, red meat is still the best source of readily absorbed iron, zinc and B vitamins. Meat today is much leaner than it used to be, and it fits the profile for a healthy diet if it is cooked with low-fat cooking methods.

Fats and Oils: Stick to low-fat products like yogurt and skim or low-fat milk, not just for a healthier, general reduction in fat intake, but also because fats require more oxygen for their metabolism and are therefore a constant drain on the body's resources.

A moderate intake of fats and oils is essential – they provide vitamins A

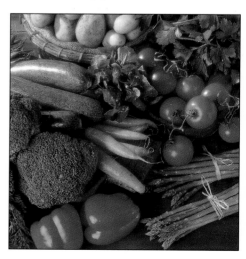

Above: Many fresh vegetables also provide beta-carotene and all are rich in fiber.

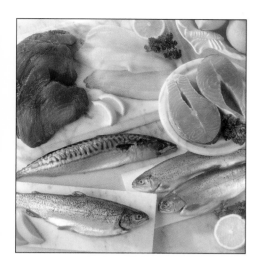

Above: A variety of oily and white fish, such as tuna, salmon and trout.

and D, and dairy products are the best source of calcium. Switch to oils high in unsaturates, like sunflower, soy, safflower, corn and olive oil – the mainstay of the Mediterranean diet – and reserve butter for special occasions when flavor really counts.

Garlic: This is reputed to have all kinds of health benefits, including helping to increase overall strength and vitality and reducing lethargy. Use it fresh or cooked, in salads, dressings and main dishes.

Nuts and Seeds: Nuts are an excellent source of protein, particularly for vegetarians. They are rich in B-group and E vitamins and provide many minerals, especially iron, zinc and potassium. Pumpkin, sunflower and sesame seeds are also rich in vitamin E and calcium. However, nuts and seeds have a high oil content (although mainly unsaturated) so watch the calories.

COOKING FOR VITALITY
Eat as much raw food as possible. Vitamins B and C are particularly unstable and are easily destroyed by heat, so include plenty of salads in your diet. Use really fresh produce, and prepare just before eating. Keep a well-stocked fruit bowl for between-meal nibbles.

Cook vegetables in a very small amount of water or steam them. Reserve any cooking water to add to soups, stews and sauces.

Trim all visible fat from meat and remove skin from poultry. If the skin is required to keep the flesh succulent, remove after cooking.

Choose low-fat cooking methods, such as broiling, stir-frying, steaming, poaching, stewing, baking and microwaving, wherever possible.

Use the minimum amount of oil for cooking and choose a type that is low in saturated fats, like olive oil or sunflower oil.

Substitute low-fat yogurt, low-fat ricotta or fat-free sour cream for cream and use reduced-fat cheeses. Parmesan and other strong-tasting cheeses are useful because you only need to use a little for a lot of flavor.

Even if you are not a vegetarian, aim to have a vegetarian meal once or twice a week. Alternatively, try to use less meat in dishes and make up the quantity with dried beans and fresh or frozen vegetables.

THE IMPORTANCE OF EXERCISE
Any form of aerobic exercise increases your intake of oxygen and improves your circulation, making the heart and

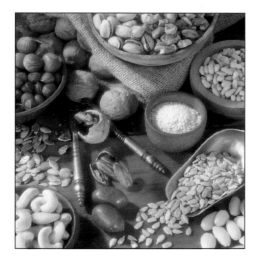

Above: Nuts and seeds not only provide essential B vitamins, minerals and protein, they also make a tasty treat.

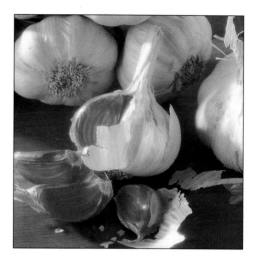

Above: Garlic is beneficial in helping to maintain good health.

all the muscles work more efficiently. Exercise creates a feeling of well-being and is wonderful for relieving stress and fatigue. It doesn't particularly matter how you choose to exercise, but pick something you enjoy, do it on a regular basis and don't overexert yourself.

BONUS HEALTH BENEFITS
Following a high vitality diet will automatically help you to control a desirable weight. Calorie counts have been included on the recipes for reference, but if you choose the right balance of foods, and take regular exercise, your weight should reach a healthy level without dieting. This will help protect you against common health risks, such as coronary heart disease, certain cancers, high blood pressure, strokes, diabetes and arthritis, all of which can be attributed to an unhealthy diet.

Reducing fat intake is of particular importance. Aim to have a total fat intake of no more than 30% of your daily calories. That should work out at between 70g and 90g a day.

Eat plenty of vitamin- and mineral-rich foods and see how your skin becomes clearer and your hair shinier. In fact, you can look forward to looking and feeling wonderful.

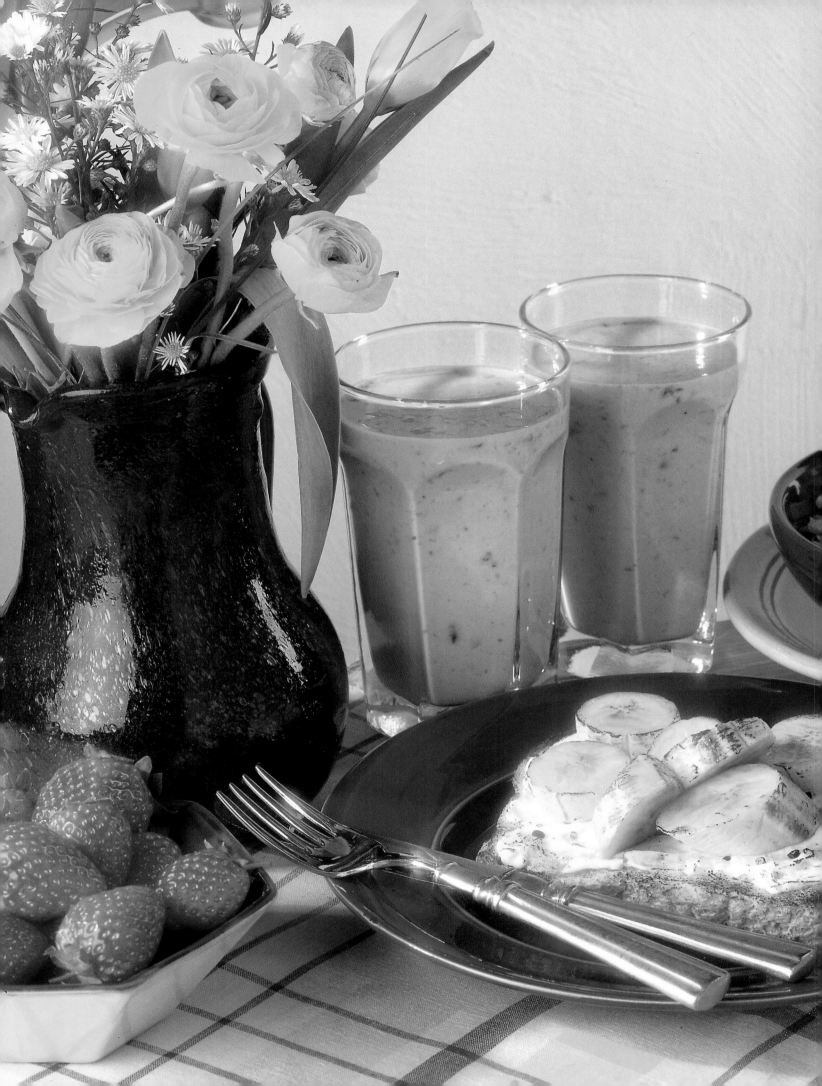

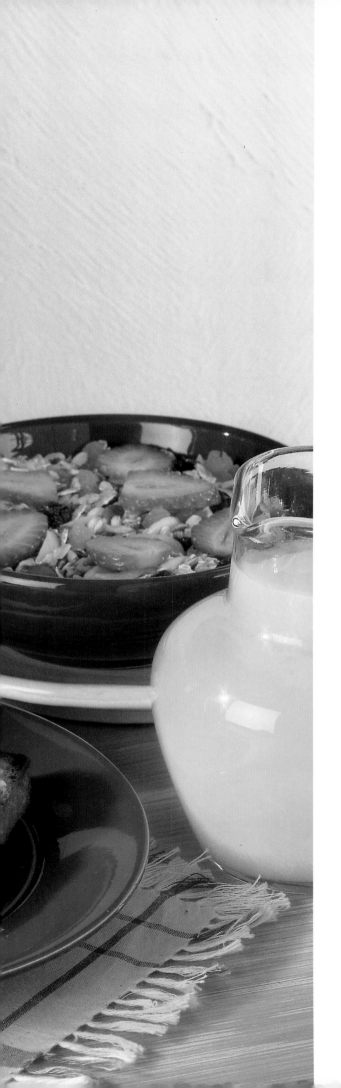

BREAKFASTS AND BRUNCHES

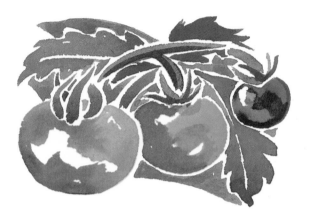

A good start in the morning is essential if you want to feel vital and alert the whole day through. Don't make the excuse of not having enough time. All the ideas here are quick to prepare and eat, yet sustaining and full of nutritional value to keep your energy levels well topped up and hunger at bay. Skip breakfast, and you're likely to succumb to far less nutritious mid-morning snacks.

Melon, Pineapple and Grape Cocktail

A light fresh fruit salad, with no
added sugar, makes a refreshing
start to the day, and can easily be
prepared the night before.

INGREDIENTS

Serves 4
½ melon
8 ounces fresh pineapple, or 8-ounce
  can pineapple chunks in own juice
8 ounces seedless white grapes, halved
½ cup white grape juice
fresh mint leaves, to decorate (optional)

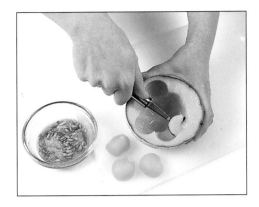

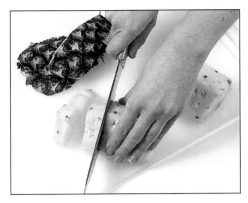

1 Remove the seeds from the melon
half and use a melon baller to
scoop out even-size balls.

2 Using a sharp knife, cut the skin
from the pineapple and discard.
Cut the fruit into bite-size chunks.

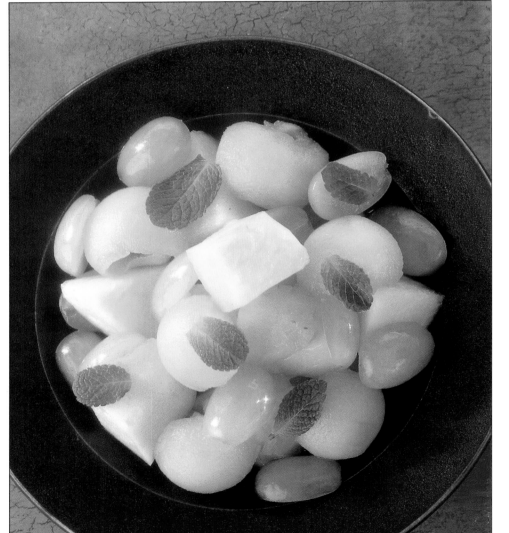

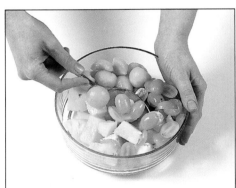

3 Combine all the fruits in a glass
serving dish and pour over the
juice. If you are using canned
pineapple, measure the drained juice
and make it up to the required quantity
with grape juice.

4 If not serving immediately, cover
and chill. Serve decorated with
mint leaves, if liked.

NUTRITIONAL NOTES	
Per Serving	
Energy	95 calories
Fat	0.5g
Saturated Fat	0
Cholesterol	0

Three Fruit Compôtes

INGREDIENTS

Each Compôte Serves 1

Orange and Prune Compôte
1 juicy orange, peeled
⅓ cup dried prunes
5 tablespoons orange juice

Pear and Kiwi Fruit Compôte
1 ripe eating pear, cored
1 kiwi fruit
4 tablespoons apple or pineapple juice

**Grapefruit and Strawberry
  Compôte**
1 grapefruit, peeled
4 ounces strawberries
4 tablespoons orange juice

To serve
plain yogurt and toasted hazelnuts

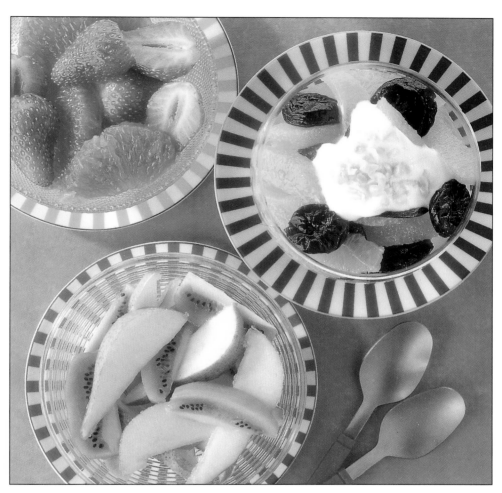

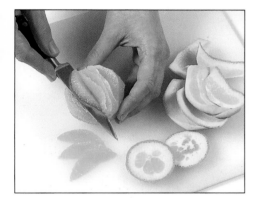

1 For the orange and prune
compôte, segment the orange and
place in a bowl with the prunes.

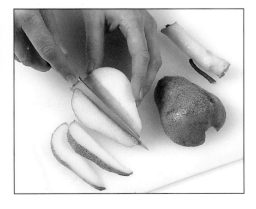

2 For the pear and kiwi fruit
compôte, slice the pear. Peel and
cut the kiwi fruit into wedges.

3 For the grapefruit and strawberry
compôte, segment the grapefruit
and halve the strawberries.

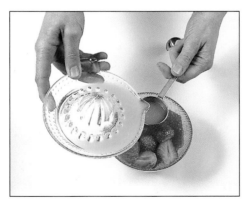

4 Place your selected fruits together
in a bowl and pour over the juice.
Choose "fresh squeezed" juices rather
than those made from concentrates.
Or, squeeze your own juice using a
blender or food processor.

5 Serve the chosen compôte topped
with a spoonful of low-fat plain
yogurt together with a sprinkling of
chopped toasted hazelnuts.

NUTRITIONAL NOTES
Per Serving (without topping)

Orange and Prune Compôte
Energy   155 calories
Fat   0.5g

Pear and Kiwi Fruit Compôte
Energy   100 calories
Fat   0.5g

Grapefruit and Strawberry Compôte
Energy   110 calories
Fat   0.5g

Neither saturated fat nor cholesterol is
present in any of the compôtes.

Date, Banana and Walnut Yogurt

Dates and bananas give a high fiber boost to this breakfast dish. Both fruits are also high in natural sugars.

INGREDIENTS

Serves 4
²/₃ cup dried dates, pitted and chopped
1¼ cups low-fat plain yogurt
2 bananas
½ cup chopped walnuts

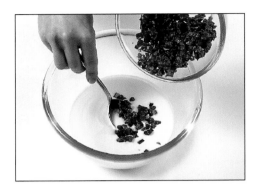

1 Stir the dates into the yogurt in a mixing bowl. Cover and leave overnight in the fridge, to allow the fruit to soften.

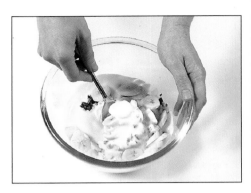

2 Peel, then slice the bananas into the yogurt mixture. Spoon into dishes and top with the walnuts.

COOK'S TIP

Use standard dried dates and not those which have been sugared. Bananas are probably the best and most convenient instant-energy food there is. If you haven't got time for breakfast, just unzip a banana!

NUTRITIONAL NOTES
Per Serving

Energy	225 calories
Fat	9.5g
Saturated Fat	1.5g
Cholesterol	3mg

Mixed Berry Yogurt Shake

Blend this in a blender or food processor for a quick, low-fat and high vitality breakfast in a glass. Rosewater adds an exotic touch. You could also experiment with other fruits to create your own flavor shake, such as banana with vanilla extract, or apricot with a few drops of almond extract.

INGREDIENTS

Serves 2
1 cup low-fat milk, chilled
1 cup low-fat plain yogurt
4 ounces mixed summer fruits
1 teaspoon rosewater
a little honey, to taste

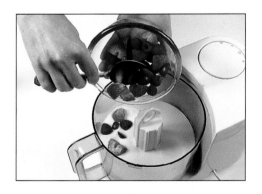

1 Blend the milk, yogurt, fruits and rosewater in a food processor.

NUTRITIONAL NOTES
Per Serving

Energy	125 calories
Fat	3.5g
Saturated Fat	2g
Cholesterol	14mg

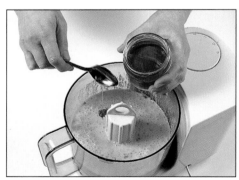

2 Add honey to taste if necessary, depending on the sweetness of the fruits. Pour into two glasses.

COOK'S TIP

Any combination of soft red fruits can be used, such as strawberries, raspberries, bilberries, blackberries, red cherries and/or red currants.

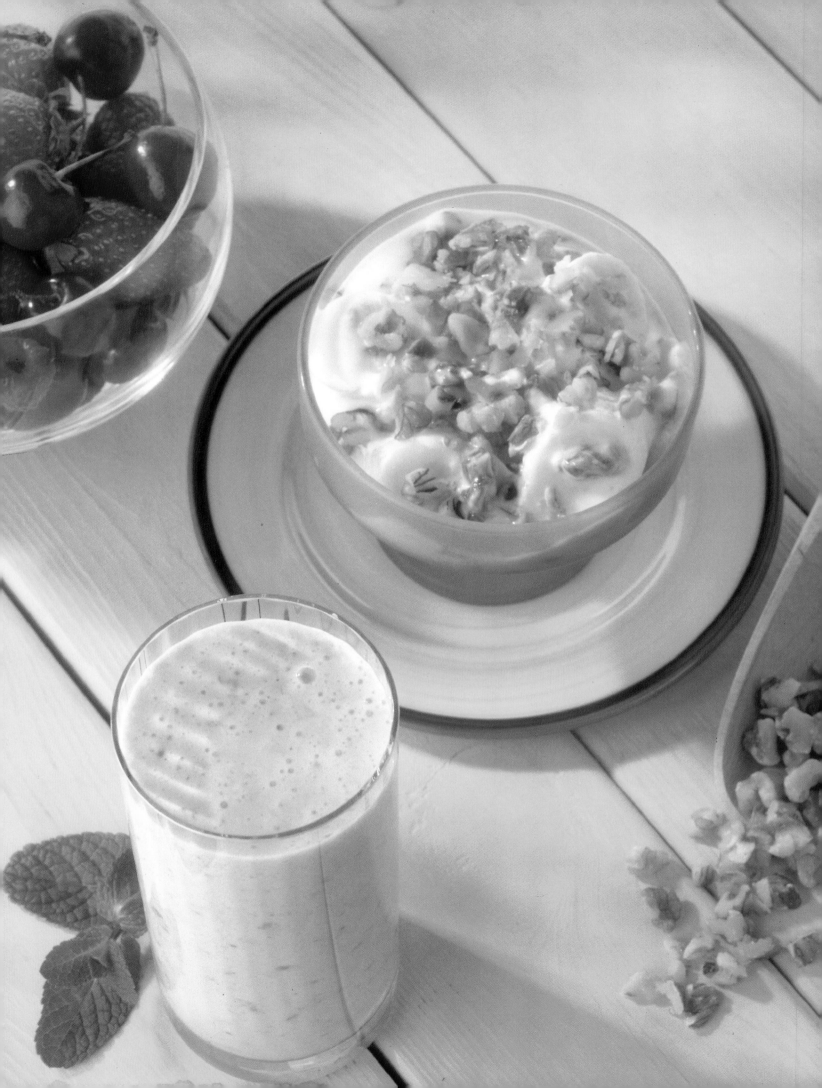

Cheese and Banana Toasties

Whole wheat toast topped with low-fat soft cheese and sliced banana makes the perfect high-fiber breakfast and is especially delicious when drizzled with honey and broiled. It's easy to make, and provides a delicious start to any day.

INGREDIENTS

Serves 4

4 thick slices of whole wheat bread
½ cup low-fat soft cream cheese
¼ teaspoon cardamom seeds, crushed (optional)
4 small bananas, peeled
4 teaspoons honey

1 Place the bread on a rack in a broiler pan and toast on one side only.

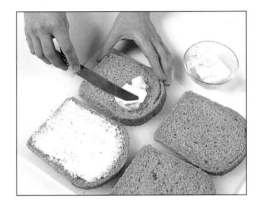

2 Turn the bread over, and spread the untoasted side of each slice with soft cheese. Sprinkle over the crushed cardamom seeds, if using.

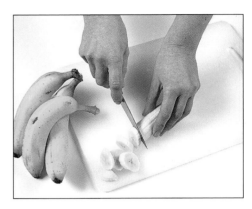

3 Slice the bananas and arrange the slices on top of the cheese. Then drizzle each slice with 1 teaspoon of the honey. Slide the pan back under the moderately hot broiler and leave for a few minutes until bubbling. Serve immediately.

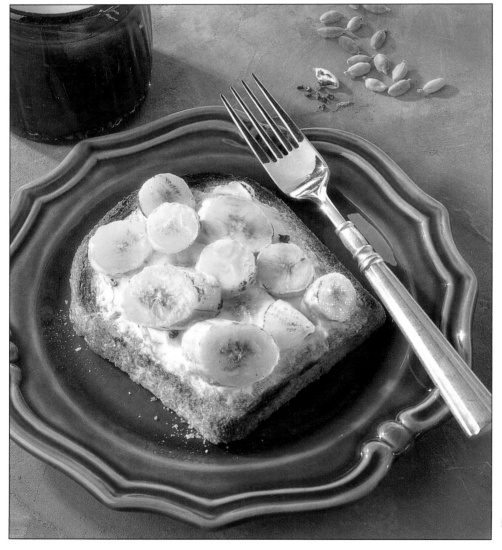

COOK'S TIP

For a delicious variation, use whole wheat bread with fruit or sesame or caraway seeds. Omit the cardamom seeds and sprinkle ground cinnamon on the bananas before adding the honey.

NUTRITIONAL NOTES
Per Serving

Energy	240 calories
Fat	4.5g
Saturated Fat	2g
Cholesterol	4mg

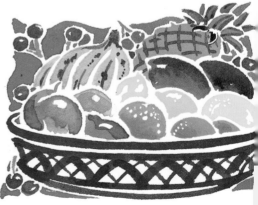

Mixed Pepper Pipérade

INGREDIENTS

Serves 4

2 tablespoons olive oil
1 onion, chopped
1 red bell pepper
1 green bell pepper
4 tomatoes, peeled and chopped
1 garlic clove, crushed
4 large eggs, beaten with 1 tablespoon
  water
ground black pepper
4 large, thick slices of whole wheat
  toast, to serve

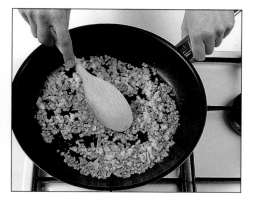

1 Heat the oil in a large frying pan and sauté the onion gently until it becomes softened.

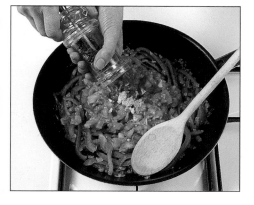

2 Remove the seeds from the red and green peppers and slice them thinly. Stir the pepper slices into the onion and cook together gently for 5 minutes. Add the tomatoes and garlic, season with black pepper, and cook for another 5 minutes.

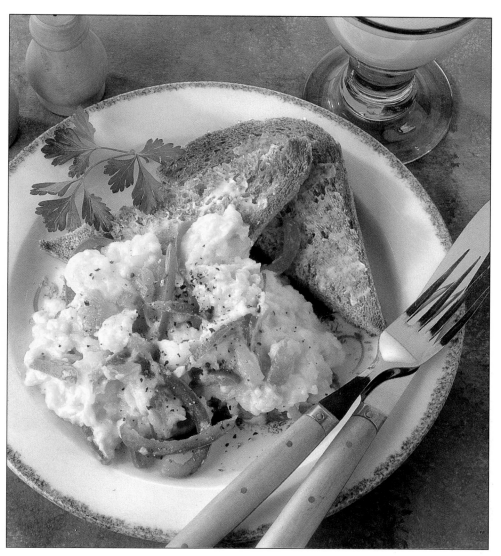

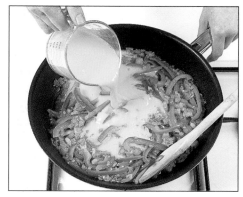

3 Pour the egg mixture over the vegetables in the frying pan and cook for 2–3 minutes, stirring now and then, until the pipérade has thickened to the consistency of lightly scrambled eggs. Serve immediately with warm whole wheat toast.

COOK'S TIP

Choose eggs that have been date-stamped for freshness. Do not stir the pipérade too much or the eggs may become rubbery.

NUTRITIONAL NOTES
Per Serving

Energy	310 calories
Fat	14.5g
Saturated Fat	3g
Cholesterol	231mg

Fruit and Sesame Cereal

Hot cereal made with skim milk makes a wonderfully nourishing breakfast. Dried fruit and toasted sesame seeds make it even better, providing useful amounts of iron and magnesium.

INGREDIENTS

Serves 2
½ cup rolled oats
2 cups skim milk
½ cup mixed dried fruits, chopped
2 tablespoons sesame seeds, toasted

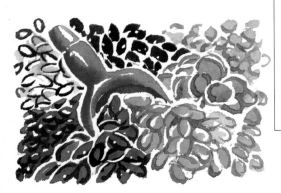

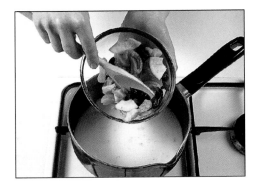

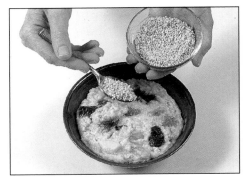

1 Put the oats, milk and chopped dried fruit in a nonstick saucepan.

2 Bring to a boil, then lower the heat and simmer gently for 3 minutes, stirring occasionally, until thickened. Serve in individual bowls, sprinkled with sesame seeds.

COOK'S TIP

If you use so-called "old-fashioned" or "original" oats, the porridge will be quite thick and coarse textured. You could also use "jumbo" oats. If you prefer a smoother porridge, try ordinary rolled oats (sometimes called oatflakes).

NUTRITIONAL NOTES	
Per Serving	
Energy	335 calories
Fat	11.5g
Saturated Fat	2g
Cholesterol	5mg

Trail Mix

Eat this nutritious snack on the run, or sprinkle it on top of yogurt or stewed fruit. It makes an excellent nibble between meals, but is quite high in calories, so don't get too carried away with it!

INGREDIENTS

Makes about 2 cups
⅓ cup dried apricots or figs, quartered
⅓ cup raisins or golden raisins
½ cup hazelnuts
scant ½ cup sunflower seeds
scant ½ cup pumpkin seeds

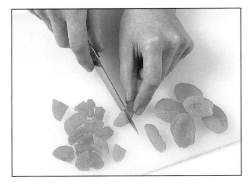

1 Cut the apricots or figs into quarters and place in a large bowl.

2 Add all the remaining ingredients and toss everything together. Store in an airtight container and use within 2–3 weeks.

COOK'S TIP

Other dried fruits or nuts may be added or substituted for those already present in the mix. Both nuts and seeds have a high oil content so will turn rancid quite quickly. To keep longer, store in the fridge.

NUTRITIONAL NOTES	
Per 1 tablespoon Serving	
Energy	70 calories
Fat	5g
Saturated Fat	1g
Cholesterol	0

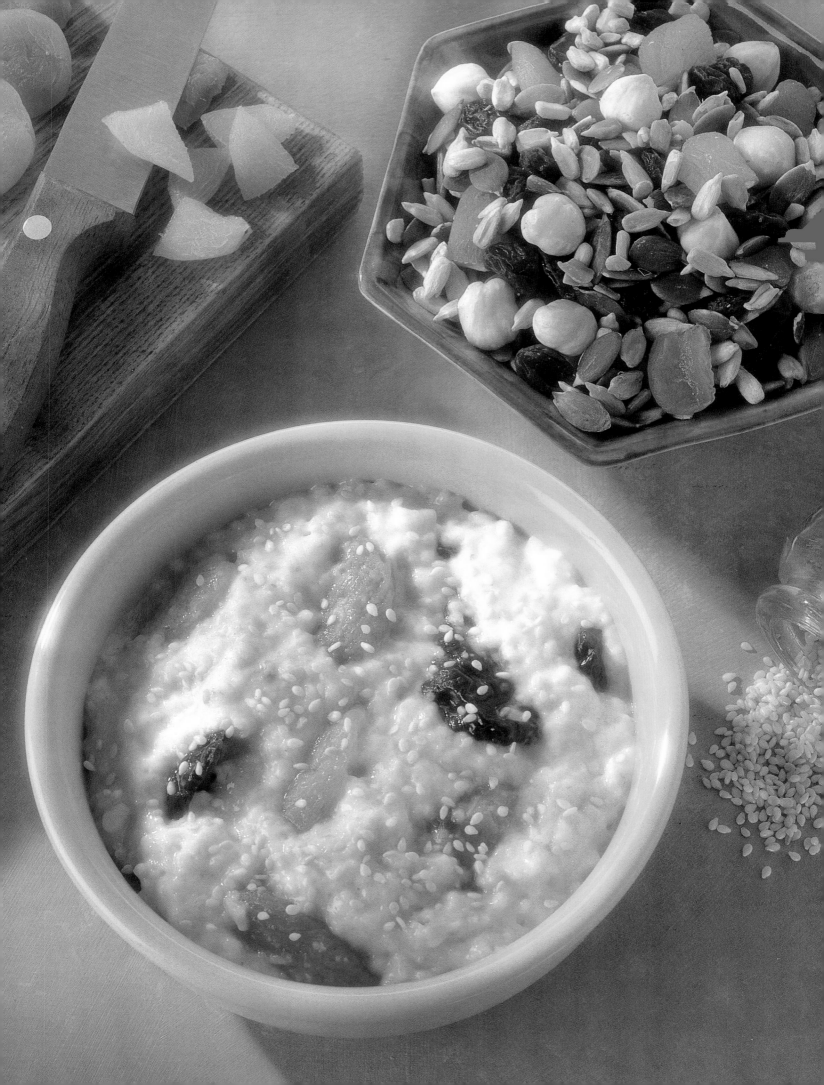

Crunchy Fruit Layer

INGREDIENTS

Serves 2

1 peach or nectarine
1 cup crunchy toasted
    oat cereal
$\frac{2}{3}$ cup low-fat plain yogurt
1 tablespoon pure fruit jam
1 tablespoon unsweetened
    fruit juice

NUTRITIONAL NOTES	
Per Serving	
Energy	240 calories
Fat	3g
Saturated Fat	1g
Cholesterol	3mg

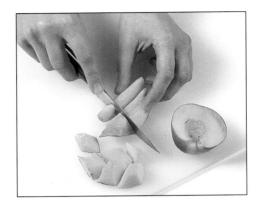

1 Remove the pit from the peach or nectarine and cut the fruit into bite-size pieces with a sharp knife.

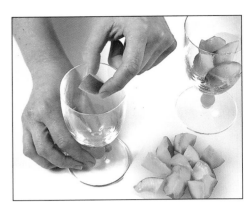

2 Divide the chopped fruit between two tall glasses, reserving a few pieces for decoration.

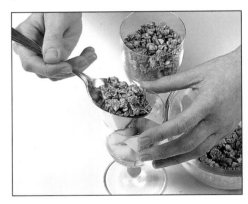

3 Sprinkle the oat cereal over the fruit in an even layer, then top with the yogurt.

4 Stir the jam and fruit juice together in a cup, then drizzle the mixture over the yogurt. Decorate with the reserved peach or nectarine and serve at once.

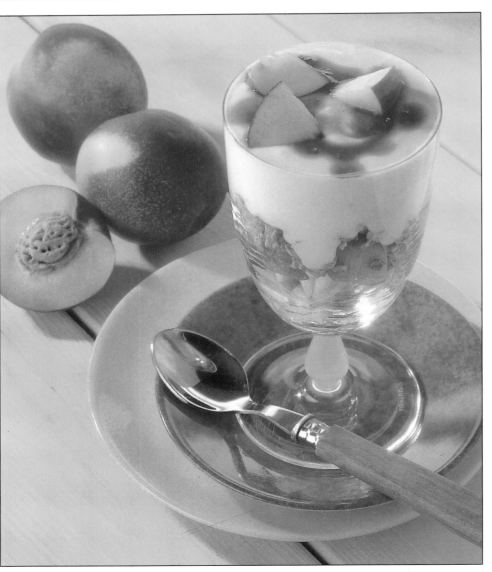

COOK'S TIP

If you prefer to use a flavored toasted oat cereal (raisin and almond, perhaps, or tropical fruits) be sure to check the nutritional information on the label and choose the variety with the lowest amount of added sugar. Any fruit jam and juice that complement each other and the chosen fruit can be used.

Apricot and Almond Muesli

There is no added sugar in this whole wheat fruit and nut muesli, which is packed with fiber, vitamins and minerals.

INGREDIENTS

Serves 8

½ cup whole blanched almonds
⅔ cup dried apricots
2 cups whole rolled oats
2 cups whole wheat flakes or
  oat bran flakes
⅓ cup raisins or golden raisins
⅓ cup pumpkin seeds
⅓ cup sunflower seeds
skim milk or low-fat plain yogurt or
  fresh fruit juice, and fresh fruit,
  to serve

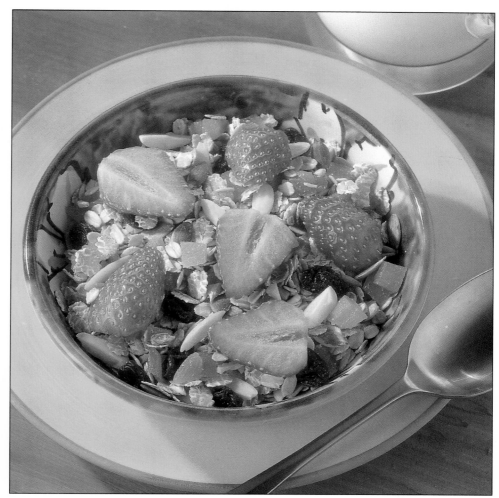

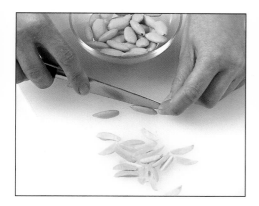

1 Using a sharp knife, carefully cut the almonds into slivers.

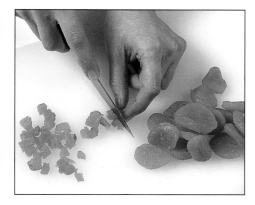

2 Cut the dried apricots into small even-size pieces.

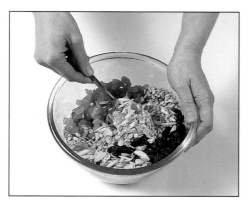

3 Stir all the ingredients together in a large bowl. Store in an airtight container and use within 6 weeks.

4 Serve with skim milk, low-fat plain yogurt or fruit juice and top with fresh fruit, such as peach, banana or strawberry slices.

--- COOK'S TIP ---

This recipe is easy to change by adding other dried fruits, such as chopped dates, figs, peaches, pear, pineapple or apple chunks. Walnuts, brazil nuts or hazelnuts could be substituted for the almonds.

NUTRITIONAL NOTES
Per Serving (without topping)

Energy	275 calories
Fat	11g
Saturated Fat	2g
Cholesterol	0

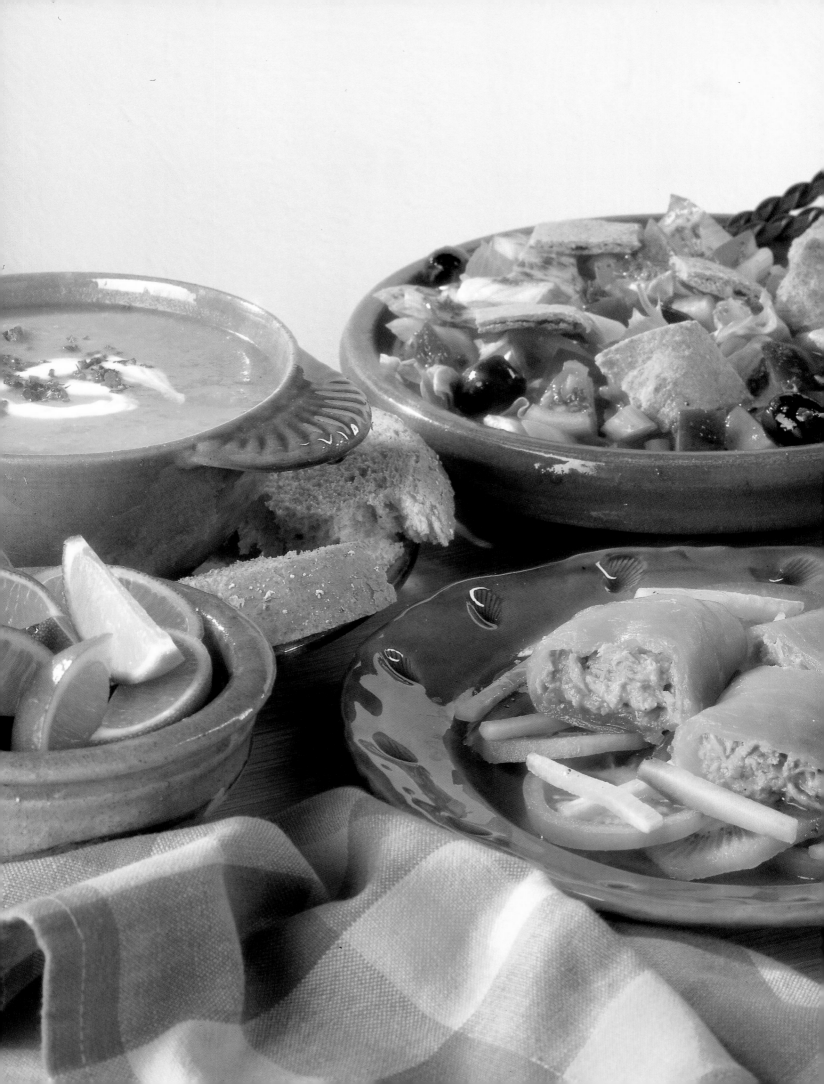

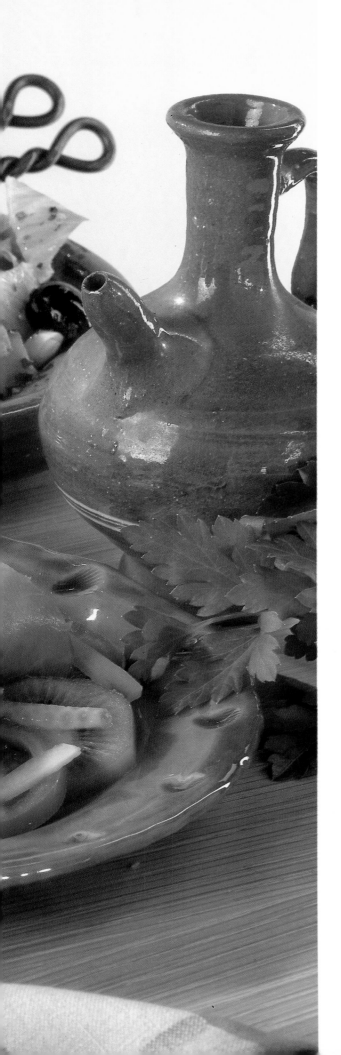

SNACKS AND LIGHT MEALS

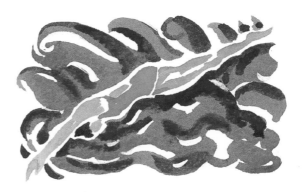

Whatever your lifestyle, whether you are out at work during the day or busy at home, there's likely to be at least one daily meal occasion when you just want something quick and easy to eat. Don't reach for a chocolate bar or pastry. The recipes in this chapter provide appetizing, yet fast ideas that are satisfying and wholesome. Home-made soup with a hunk of whole-grain bread is perfect for a snatched lunch, or try some more unusual sandwich or baked potato ideas. Go wild with exciting salad combinations, borrow inspiration from foreign cuisines and widen your appreciation of vegetarian dishes.

Spicy Tomato and Lentil Soup

INGREDIENTS

Serves 4

1 tablespoon sunflower oil
1 onion, finely chopped
1–2 garlic cloves, crushed
1-inch piece of fresh ginger, peeled and
    finely chopped
1 teaspoon cumin seeds, crushed
1 pound ripe tomatoes, peeled, seeded
    and chopped
²/₃ cup red lentils
5 cups vegetable or chicken stock
1 tablespoon tomato paste
salt and ground black pepper
low-fat plain natural yogurt and
    chopped fresh parsley, to garnish
    (optional)

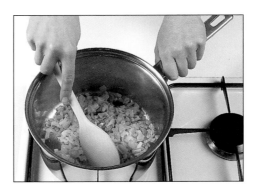

1 Heat the sunflower oil in a large heavy-bottomed saucepan and cook the chopped onion gently for about 5 minutes, until softened.

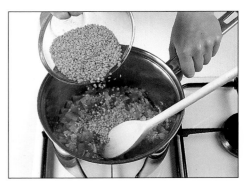

2 Stir in the garlic, ginger and cumin seeds, followed by the tomatoes and lentils. Cook over low heat for another 3–4 minutes.

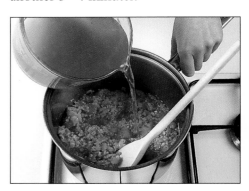

3 Stir in the stock and tomato paste. Bring to a boil, then lower the heat and simmer gently for about 30 minutes, or until the lentils are soft. Season to taste with salt and pepper.

4 Purée the soup in a blender or food processor. Return to the clean pan and reheat gently. Serve in heated bowls. Garnish each portion with a swirl of yogurt, if liked, and sprinkle over a little chopped parsley.

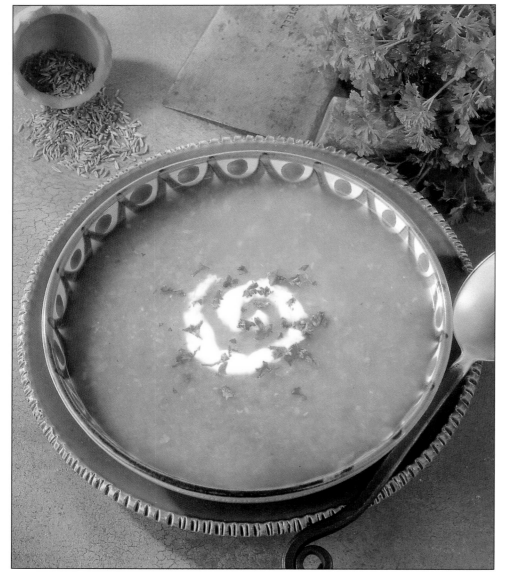

NUTRITIONAL NOTES	
Per Serving	
Energy	165 calories
Fat	4g
Saturated Fat	0.5g
Cholesterol	0

Chunky Bean and Vegetable Soup

A substantial soup, not unlike minestrone, using a selection of vegetables, with cannellini beans for extra protein and fiber. Serve with a hunk of whole wheat bread.

INGREDIENTS

Serves 4

2 tablespoons olive oil
2 celery stalks, chopped
2 leeks, sliced
3 carrots, sliced
2 garlic cloves, crushed
14-ounce can chopped tomatoes
    with basil
5 cups vegetable stock
15-ounce can cannellini beans (or
    mixed beans), drained
1 tablespoon pesto sauce
salt and ground black pepper
shavings of Parmesan cheese, to serve

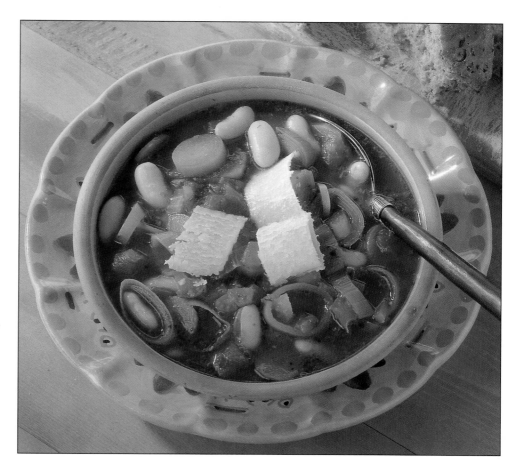

COOK'S TIP

Extra vegetables can be added to the soup to make it even more substantial. For example, add some thinly sliced zucchini or finely shredded cabbage for the last 5 minutes of the cooking time. Or, stir in some small whole wheat pasta shapes, if you like. Add them at the same time as the tomatoes, as they will take 10–15 minutes to cook.

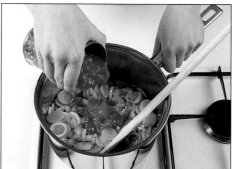

2 Stir in the tomatoes and the stock. Bring to a boil, then cover and cook gently for 15 minutes.

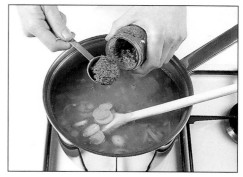

3 Stir in the beans and pesto, with salt and pepper to taste. Heat through for another 5 minutes. Serve in heated bowls, sprinkled with shavings of Parmesan cheese.

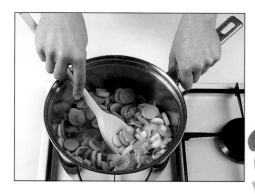

1 Heat the olive oil in a large saucepan. Add the celery, leeks, carrots and garlic and cook gently for about 5 minutes, until softened.

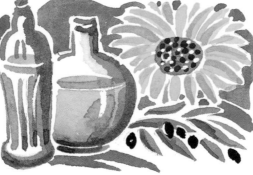

NUTRITIONAL NOTES	
Per Serving	
Energy	205 calories
Fat	11.5g
Saturated Fat	3g
Cholesterol	8.5mg

Provençal Pan Bagna

A whole wheat French stick, filled with salad and sardines, provides protein, fiber, vitamins and minerals and gives a completely new meaning to the term "brown bag lunch."

INGREDIENTS

Serves 3

1 whole wheat French stick or 3 large whole wheat rolls
2 garlic cloves, crushed
3 tablespoons olive oil
1 small onion, thinly sliced
2 tomatoes, sliced
3-inch length of cucumber, sliced
4 ounces canned sardines in tomato sauce
2 tablespoons chopped fresh parsley
ground black pepper

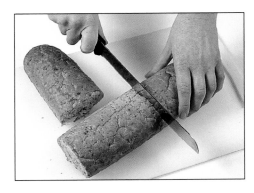

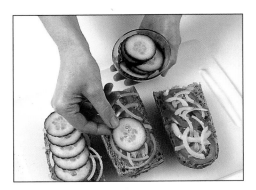

1 Cut the French stick into three equal pieces, then slice each piece in half lengthwise. If using rolls, split them in half. Squash down the soft inside of the bread to make a shallow hollow for the filling. Mix the garlic with the oil, then brush over the inside of the bread.

2 Lay slices of onion, tomato and cucumber on one half of the bread. Top with the sardines in tomato sauce. If you are concerned about the bones in the fish, you could slice open the sardines and remove the larger pieces, but it makes sound nutritional sense to leave them, as they are edible and are an excellent source of calcium.

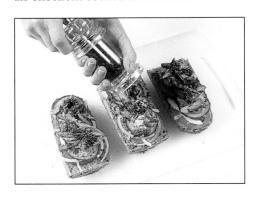

3 Sprinkle the parsley over the fish and season with pepper. Sandwich the bread halves back together and wrap tightly in foil or plastic wrap. Chill for at least 30 minutes before eating.

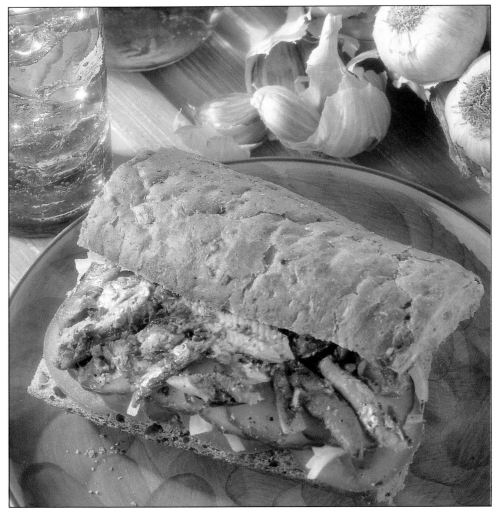

NUTRITIONAL NOTES	
Per Serving	
Energy	320 calories
Fat	17.5g
Saturated Fat	3.5g
Cholesterol	30.5mg

Guacamole Pita Pocket

Although they have a reputation for being high in fat and calories, avocados are very nutritious. The high oil content is mainly mono-unsaturated and they are rich in vitamin A.

INGREDIENTS

Serves 2

2 whole wheat pita breads
2 teaspoons Tabasco sauce or chili sauce (optional)
crisp lettuce, shredded

For the guacamole
1 large ripe avocado
juice of ½ lemon
1 garlic clove, crushed
1 tablespoon finely chopped cilantro
2 tomatoes, coarsely chopped
2-inch length of cucumber, diced
salt and ground black pepper

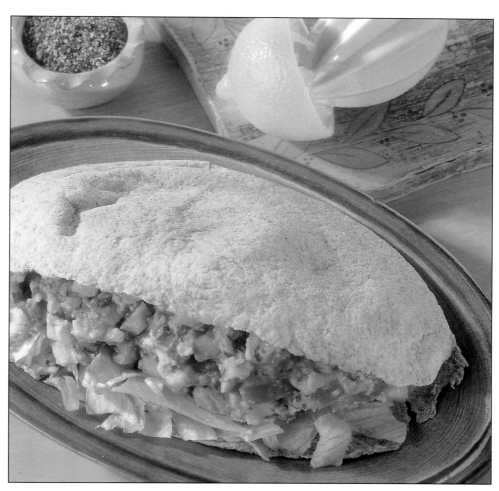

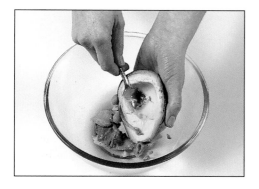

1 Make the guacamole. Cut the avocado in half, remove the pit and scoop out the flesh into a bowl. Chop the flesh coarsely, sprinkle it with the lemon juice, then mash, leaving the flesh slightly chunky.

2 Stir in the garlic and cilantro. Add the tomatoes and cucumber, with salt and pepper to taste, and mix.

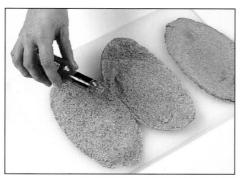

3 Warm the pita breads briefly in a warm oven or toaster, then slit them open lengthwise and open them out to reveal the pockets. Sprinkle a little Tabasco sauce or chili sauce on the inside, if liked.

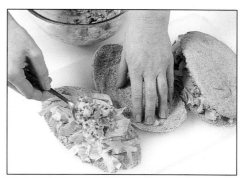

4 Half fill the pita pockets with lettuce, then spoon the guacamole on top. Serve immediately.

—————— COOK'S TIP ——————

Do not toast the pita breads – the aim is simply to refresh them.

NUTRITIONAL NOTES
Per Serving

Energy	345 calories
Fat	21g
Saturated Fat	3g
Cholesterol	0

Zucchini and Potato Tortilla

INGREDIENTS

Serves 4

1 pound potatoes, peeled and diced
2 tablespoons olive oil
1 onion, finely chopped
1 garlic clove, crushed
2 zucchini, thinly sliced
2 tablespoons chopped fresh tarragon
4 large eggs, beaten
salt and ground black pepper

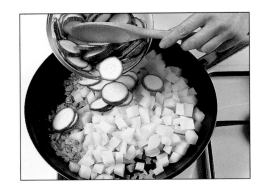

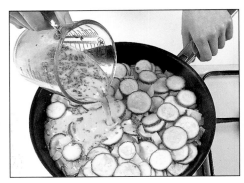

NUTRITIONAL NOTES	
Per Serving	
Energy	265 calories
Fat	14.5g
Saturated Fat	3g
Cholesterol	231mg

1 Cook the potatoes in boiling, salted water for about 5 minutes.

2 Heat the oil in a large frying pan which can also be used under the broiler. Add the onion and cook gently for 3–4 minutes, until it is beginning to soften. Add the potatoes, garlic and zucchini to the pan. Cook for about 5 minutes more, shaking the pan occasionally to prevent the potatoes from sticking to the bottom, until the zucchini are softened and the potatoes are lightly browned.

3 Stir the tarragon into the eggs and season with salt and pepper. Pour the eggs over the vegetables in the pan and cook over moderate heat until the underside of the tortilla is set. Meanwhile, preheat the broiler.

4 Place the pan under the broiler and cook for a few minutes more, until the top of the tortilla has set. Cut into wedges and serve from the pan.

Chicken and Pesto Baked Potatoes

Although it is usually served with pasta, pesto also gives a wonderful lift to rice, bread and potato dishes – all good starchy carbohydrates. Here, it is combined with chicken and yogurt to make a low-fat topping for baked potatoes.

INGREDIENTS

Serves 4

4 baking potatoes, pricked
2 boned chicken breasts
1 cup low-fat plain yogurt
1 tablespoon pesto sauce
fresh basil, to garnish

1 Preheat the oven to 400°F. Bake the potatoes for about 1¼ hours, or until they are soft on the inside when tested with a knife.

2 About 20 minutes before the potatoes are ready, cook the chicken breasts, leaving the skin on, so that the flesh remains moist. Either bake the breasts in a dish alongside the potatoes in the oven, or cook them on a rack under a moderately hot broiler.

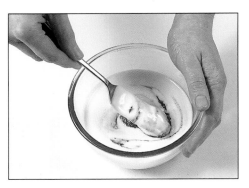

3 Stir together the yogurt and pesto. When the potatoes are cooked through, cut them open. Skin the chicken breasts.

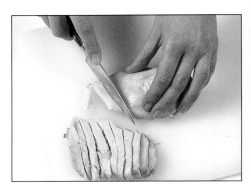

4 Slice the chicken, then fill the potatoes with the slices, top with the yogurt and garnish with basil.

NUTRITIONAL NOTES	
Per Serving	
Energy	310 calories
Fat	5.5g
Saturated Fat	1.5g
Cholesterol	35.5mg

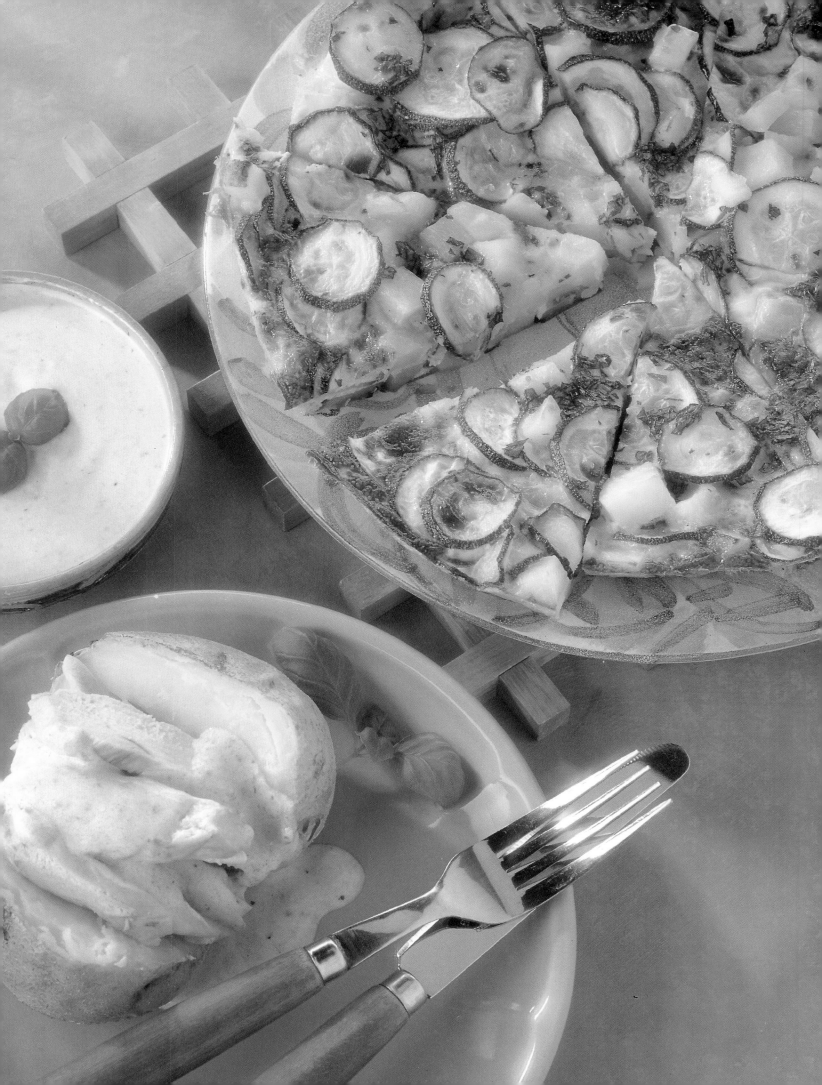

Two Pear Salad

INGREDIENTS

Serves 4
2 zucchini, grated
2 avocados
2 ripe eating pears
1 large carrot

For the dressing
1 cup low-fat plain yogurt
4 tablespoons reduced-fat mayonnaise
grated rind of 1 lemon
8 – 10 chives, chopped
2 tablespoons chopped fresh mint
ground black pepper
4 mint sprigs, to garnish

1 Pile the grated zucchini on to four individual serving plates.

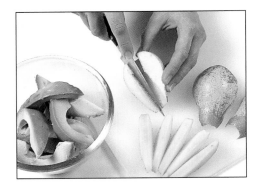

2 Cut the avocados in half, then remove the pits and peel. Slice each half lengthwise. Core and slice the pears. Arrange avocado and pear slices on top of each zucchini salad.

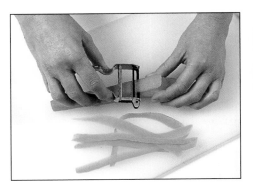

3 Peel the carrot, then use the peeler to peel off fine ribbons.

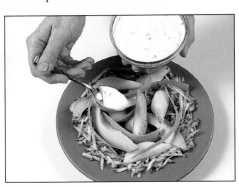

4 Make the dressing. Mix the yogurt and mayonnaise together in a bowl, then stir in the lemon rind, chives and chopped mint. Season with pepper. Drizzle some of the dressing over each salad and garnish with a mint sprig. Serve immediately.

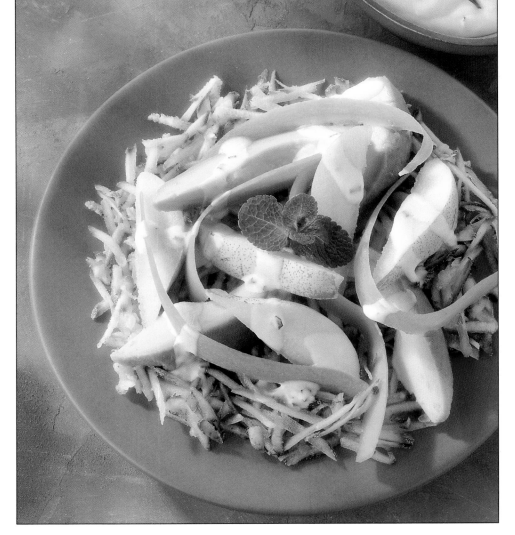

COOK'S TIP

If the salad is not to be served right away, sprinkle the avocado with lemon juice or the flesh will discolor.

NUTRITIONAL NOTES
Per Serving

Energy	260 calories
Fat	19.5g
Saturated Fat	3g
Cholesterol	2.5g

Four Seasons Salad Platter

Fresh vegetable salads are packed with vitamin C. Include some protein foods and serve with a hunk of fresh whole wheat bread for a well-balanced snack or simple lunch.

INGREDIENTS

Serves 2

4 Belgian endive leaves
4 ounces green beans, lightly cooked
3-inch length of cucumber, cut into sticks
6 cherry tomatoes
1 hard-boiled egg, halved

Carrot and Radish Salad

2 carrots
2 radishes
1 tablespoon chopped mixed nuts

Beet and Onion Salad

2–3 cooked beets, sliced
1 tablespoon balsamic or wine vinegar
2–3 scallions, finely chopped
2 tablespoons chopped fresh parsley

Mushroom and Thyme Salad

³/₄ cup button mushrooms, sliced
2 tablespoons lemon juice
1 tablespoon chopped fresh thyme

Tuna and Haricot Bean Salad

3½-ounce can tuna in oil
7-ounce can navy beans
½ red onion, thinly sliced
2 tablespoons chopped fresh parsley

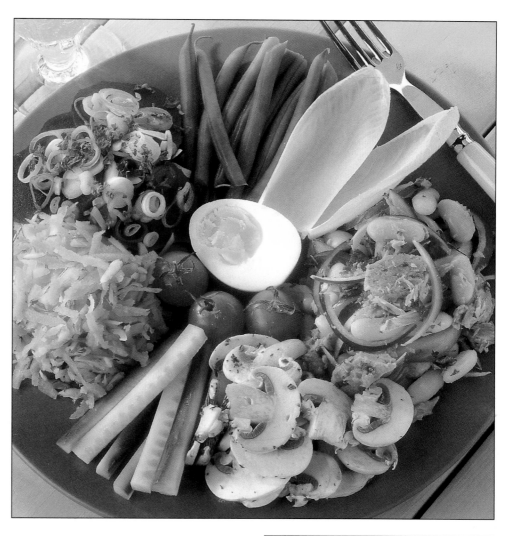

NUTRITIONAL NOTES	
Per Serving (including bread)	
Energy	405 calories
Fat	13.5g
Saturated Fat	2.5g
Cholesterol	122.5mg

1 Grate the carrots and radishes. Mix together with the nuts in a bowl.

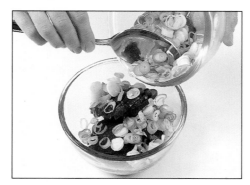

2 Sprinkle the beets with vinegar, add the scallions and parsley and toss lightly.

3 Mix the mushrooms with the lemon juice and thyme.

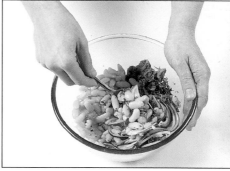

4 Drain the tuna and beans, turn them both into a bowl and toss with the onion and parsley.

5 Divide the Belgian endive leaves between two large salad plates. Add a portion of each salad, arranging them attractively with the green beans, cucumber sticks, tomatoes and egg halves. Serve with whole wheat bread.

Stuffed Vine Leaves

Based on the Greek *dolmas* (or *dolmades*) but with a whole-grain vegetarian stuffing, this makes an excellent low-fat, high-fiber appetizer, snack or buffet dish.

INGREDIENTS

Makes about 40

1 tablespoon sunflower oil
1 teaspoon sesame oil
1 onion, finely chopped
1⅓ cups brown rice
2½ cups vegetable stock
1 small yellow bell pepper, seeded and finely chopped
⅔ cup dried apricots, finely chopped
2 lemons
½ cup pine nuts
3 tablespoons chopped fresh parsley
2 tablespoons chopped fresh mint
½ teaspoon mixed spice
8-ounce jar vine leaves preserved in brine, drained
2 tablespoons olive oil
ground black pepper
lemon wedges, to garnish

To serve

1¼ cups low-fat plain yogurt
2 tablespoons chopped fresh mixed herbs
cayenne pepper

COOK'S TIP

If vine leaves are not available, the leaves of Swiss chard, young spinach or cabbage can be used instead.

NUTRITIONAL NOTES
Per Stuffed Vine Leaf

Energy	45 calories
Fat	2g
Saturated Fat	0.5g
Cholesterol	trace

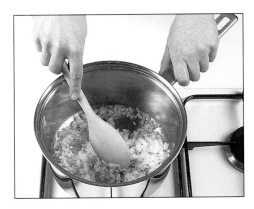

1 Heat the sunflower and sesame oils together in a fairly large saucepan. Add the onion and cook gently for 5 minutes to soften.

2 Add the rice, stirring to coat the grains in oil. Pour in the stock, bring to a boil, then lower the heat, cover the pan and simmer for about 30 minutes, or until the rice is tender but retains a little "bite."

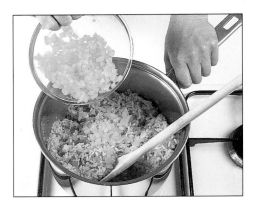

3 Stir in the chopped pepper and apricots, with a little more stock if necessary. Replace the lid and cook for another 5 minutes.

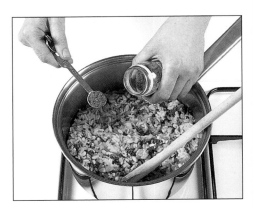

4 Grate 1 lemon, then squeeze both lemons. Drain off any stock which has not been absorbed by the rice. Stir in the pine nuts, herbs, mixed spice, lemon rind and half the juice. Season with pepper and set aside.

5 Bring a saucepan of water to a boil and blanch the vine leaves for about 5 minutes. Drain the leaves well, then lay them shiny side down on a board. Cut out any coarse stalks.

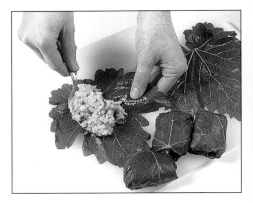

6 Place a heap of the rice mixture in the center of each vine leaf. Fold the stem end over, then the sides and pointed end to make neat packages. Pack the packages closely together in a shallow serving dish. Mix the remaining lemon juice with the olive oil. Pour the mixture over the vine leaves, cover and chill before serving. Garnish with lemon wedges. Spoon the yogurt into a bowl, stir in the chopped herbs and sprinkle with a little cayenne. Serve with the stuffed vine leaves.

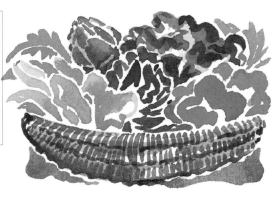

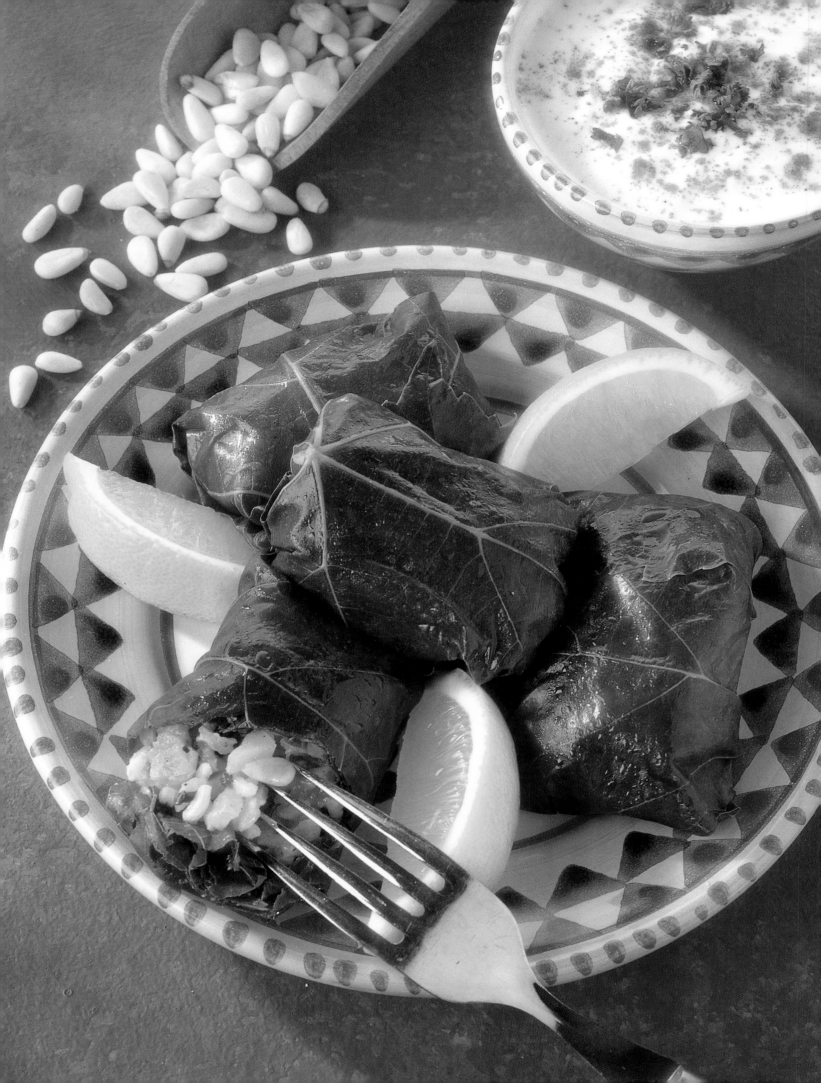

Mango, Shrimp and Tomato Vinaigrette

INGREDIENTS

Serves 4

1 large mango
8 ounces cooked shrimp, peeled and
  deveined
16 cherry tomatoes, halved
fresh mint sprigs, to garnish

For the dressing
1 tablespoon white wine vinegar
½ teaspoon honey
1 tablespoon mango or apricot chutney
1 tablespoon chopped fresh mint
1 tablespoon chopped fresh lemon
  balm
3 tablespoons olive oil

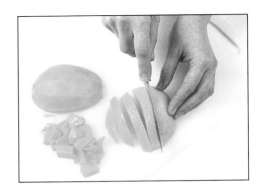

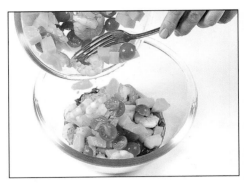

1 Using a sharp knife, peel, pit and dice the mango carefully. Mix with the shrimp and cherry tomatoes in a bowl. Toss lightly to mix, then cover and chill.

2 Make the salad dressing by mixing the vinegar, honey, chutney and fresh herbs in a bowl. Gradually whisk in the olive oil, then add salt and pepper to taste.

3 Spoon the shrimp mixture into the dressing and toss lightly, then divide among serving dishes. Garnish with the fresh mint sprigs and serve.

NUTRITIONAL NOTES
Per Serving

Energy	230 calories
Fat	10g
Saturated Fat	1.5g
Cholesterol	45.5mg

COOK'S TIP

If you use frozen shrimp, thaw them in a strainer, then drain thoroughly on paper towels before use or the water will dilute the salad dressing and spoil the flavor.

Chicken Salad with Cranberry Dressing

INGREDIENTS

Serves 4

4 boned chicken breasts, total weight
  about 1½ pounds
1¼ cups stock or a mixture of stock
  and white wine
fresh herb sprigs
7 ounces mixed salad leaves
½ cup chopped walnuts
  or hazelnuts

For the dressing
2 tablespoons olive oil
1 tablespoon walnut or hazelnut oil
1 tablespoon raspberry or red
  wine vinegar
2 tablespoons cranberry relish
salt and ground black pepper

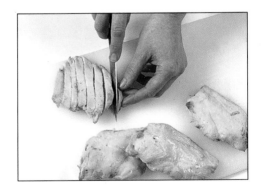

1 Skin the chicken breasts. Pour the stock (or stock and wine mixture) into a large shallow saucepan. Add the herbs and bring the liquid to simmering point. Poach the chicken breasts for about 15 minutes, until cooked through. Alternatively, leave the skin on the breasts and broil or roast them until tender, then remove the skin.

2 Arrange the salad leaves on four plates. Slice each chicken breast neatly, keeping the slices together, then place each breast on top of a portion of salad, fanning the slices out slightly.

3 Make the dressing by shaking all the ingredients together in a screw-top jar. Spoon a little dressing over each salad and sprinkle with the walnuts or hazelnuts.

NUTRITIONAL NOTES
Per Serving

Energy	365 calories
Fat	22g
Saturated Fat	3.5g
Cholesterol	64.5mg

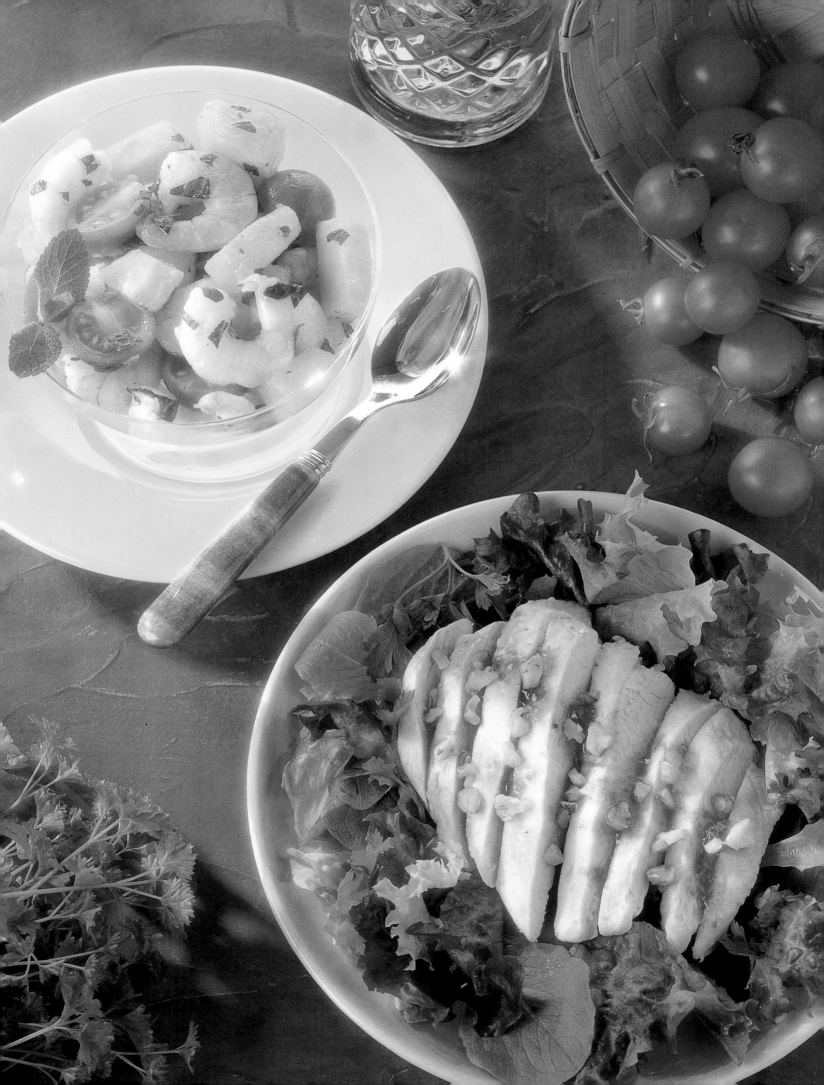

Mushroom, Leek and Cashew Risotto

INGREDIENTS

Serves 4

1⅓ cups brown rice

3¾ cups vegetable stock or a mixture of stock and dry white wine in the ratio of 5 to 1

1 tablespoon walnut or hazelnut oil

2 leeks, sliced

2 cups mixed wild or cultivated mushrooms, trimmed and sliced

½ cup cashew nuts

grated rind of 1 lemon

2 tablespoons chopped fresh thyme

scant ¼ cup pumpkin seeds

salt and ground black pepper

fresh thyme leaves and lemon wedges, to garnish

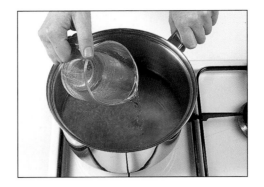

1 Place the brown rice in a large saucepan, pour in the vegetable stock (or stock and wine), and bring to a boil. Lower the heat and cook gently for about 30 minutes, until all the stock has been absorbed and the rice grains are tender.

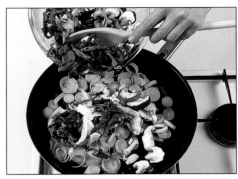

2 About 6 minutes before the rice is cooked, heat the oil in a large frying pan, add the sliced leeks and mushrooms and fry over gentle heat for 3 – 4 minutes.

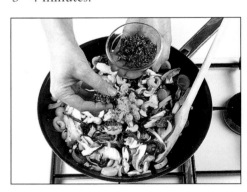

3 Add the cashew nuts, lemon rind and chopped thyme to the vegetables and cook for 1 – 2 minutes more. Season with salt and pepper.

4 Drain off any excess stock from the cooked rice and stir in the vegetable mixture. Turn into a serving dish. Sprinkle the pumpkin seeds over the top and garnish with the fresh thyme sprigs and lemon wedges. Serve at once.

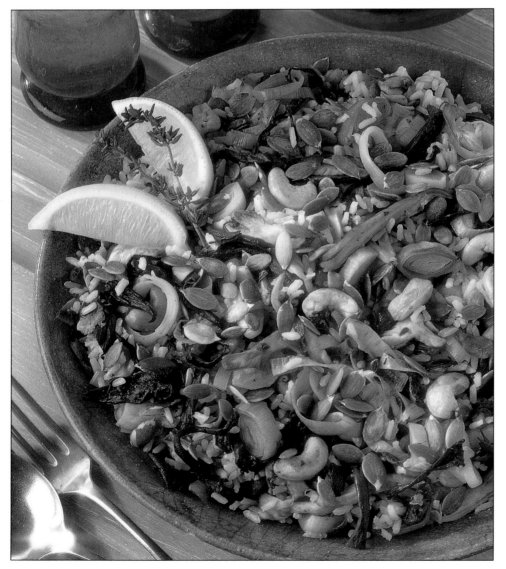

NUTRITIONAL NOTES	
Per Serving	
Energy	395 calories
Fat	14g
Saturated Fat	2.5g
Cholesterol	0

Fattoush

This Middle-Eastern mixed salad is traditionally topped with pieces of unleavened bread to soak up the dressing. It provides the perfect solution of what to do with slightly stale pita breads.

INGREDIENTS

Serves 4

2 whole wheat pita breads
1 iceberg or Romaine lettuce, torn
   into pieces
1 green bell pepper, seeded
4-inch length of cucumber
4 tomatoes
4 scallions
a few black olives, to garnish

For the dressing

4 tablespoons olive oil
3 tablespoons freshly squeezed
   lemon juice
2 garlic cloves, crushed
3 tablespoons finely chopped
   fresh parsley
2 tablespoons finely chopped fresh mint
few drops of harissa or chili sauce
   (optional)
salt and ground black pepper

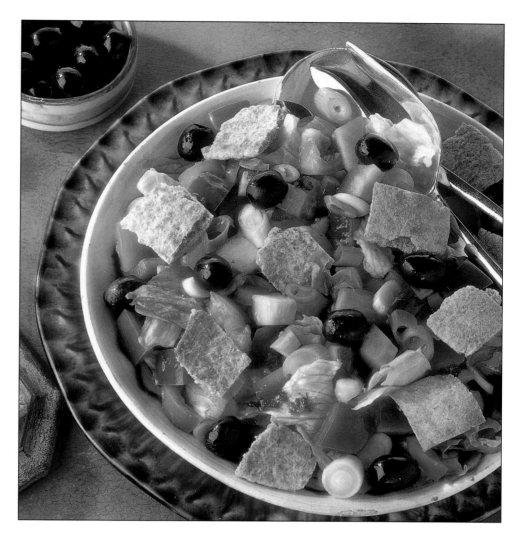

------ COOK'S TIP ------

Any green leaves can be used instead of lettuce. Try young spinach leaves or mesclun for a change.

2 Place the lettuce in a large bowl. Chop the green pepper, cucumber, tomatoes and scallions coarsely, making sure they are all about the same size. Add them to the lettuce and toss together well.

4 Just before serving the dish, pour the dressing from the jar over the salad and toss well to combine together. Sprinkle pieces of pita bread over the salad and garnish with the black olives.

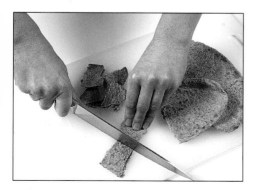

1 Broil or toast the pita breads on both sides until crisp and golden. Cut into rough squares and set aside.

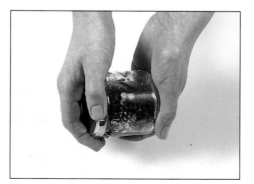

3 Make the dressing by shaking all the ingredients together in a screw-top jar.

NUTRITIONAL NOTES
Per Serving

Energy	225 calories
Fat	13g
Saturated Fat	2g
Cholesterol	0

Salmon and Tuna Packages

You need fairly large smoked salmon slices as they are wrapped around a light tuna mixture before being served on a vibrant salad. Kiwi fruit is a particularly rich source of Vitamin C.

INGREDIENTS

Serves 4
2 tablespoons low-fat plain yogurt
1 tablespoon sun-dried tomato paste
1 teaspoon whole-grain honey mustard
grated rind and juice of 1 lime
7-ounce can tuna in water, drained
4½ ounces smoked salmon slices
ground black pepper
fresh mint leaves, to garnish

For the salad
3 tomatoes, sliced
2 kiwi fruit, peeled and sliced
¼ cucumber, cut into julienne sticks
1 tablespoon chopped fresh mint
3 tablespoons vinaigrette dressing

COOK'S TIP

Although healthy eating guidelines recommend reducing the amount of fat (particularly saturated fat) in the diet, salad dressings made with polyunsaturated or monounsaturated oil, such as olive oil, can and should be included, in sensible moderation. This recipe is not high in calories, but if weight control is a real issue, use an oil-free dressing instead of vinaigrette.

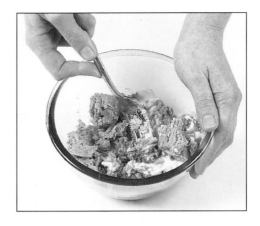

1 Mix the yogurt, tomato paste and mustard in a bowl. Stir in the grated lime rind and juice. Add the tuna, with black pepper to taste, and mix well.

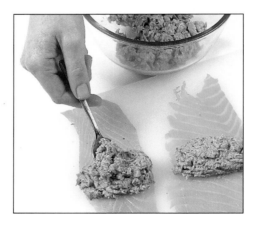

2 Spread out the salmon slices on a board and spoon some of the tuna mixture on to each piece.

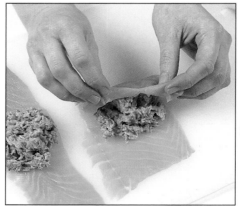

3 Roll up or fold the smoked salmon into neat packages. Carefully press the edges together to seal.

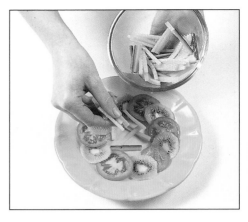

4 Make the salad. Arrange the tomato and kiwi slices on four serving plates. Sprinkle over the cucumber sticks. Add the chopped mint to the vinaigrette dressing and spoon a little over each salad.

5 Arrange 3–4 salmon packages on each salad, garnish with the mint leaves and serve.

NUTRITIONAL NOTES
Per Serving

Energy	200 calories
Fat	11.5g
Saturated Fat	2g
Cholesterol	33.5mg

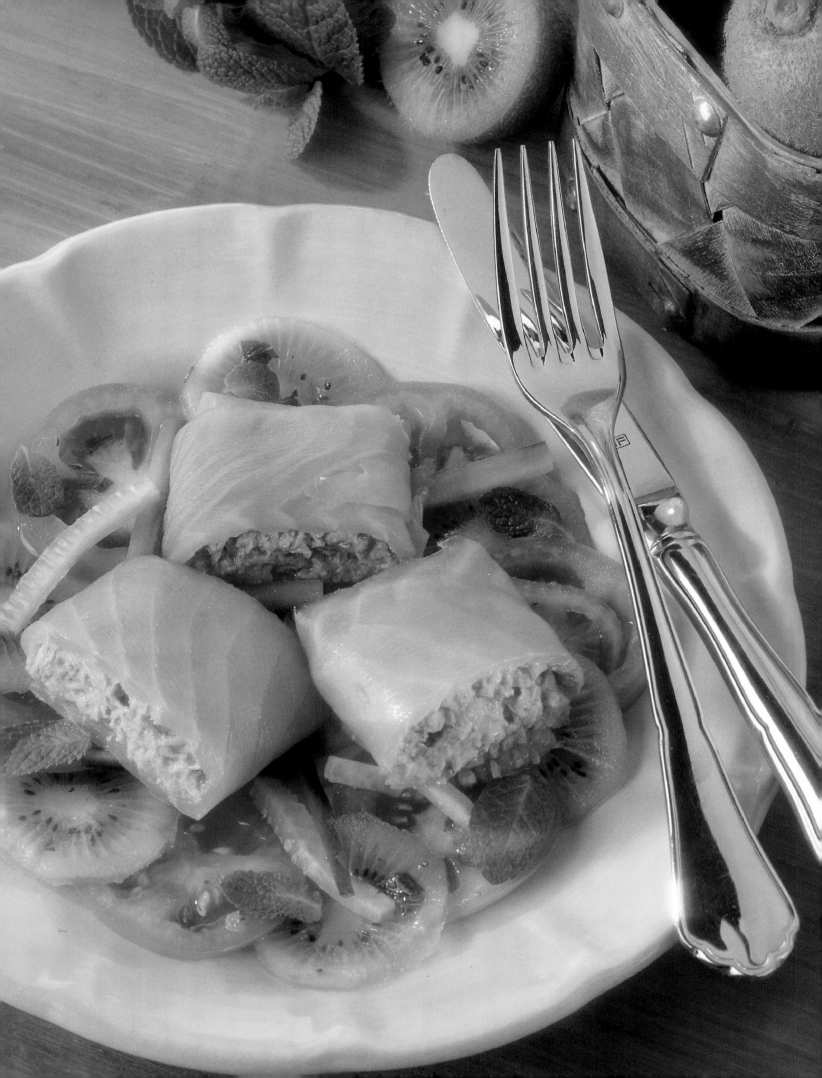

Eggs en Cocotte

INGREDIENTS

Serves 4

4 eggs
4 teaspoons freshly grated
   Parmesan cheese
chopped fresh parsley, to garnish

For the ratatouille

1 small red bell pepper
1 tablespoon olive oil
1 onion, finely chopped
1 garlic clove, crushed
2 zucchini, diced
14-ounce can chopped tomatoes
   with basil
salt and ground black pepper

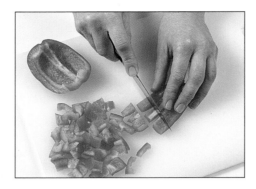

1 Using a sharp vegetable knife, cut the red pepper in half on a board and remove the seeds. Then cut the red pepper into dice. Preheat the oven to 375°F.

2 Heat the oil in a frying pan. Add the onion, garlic, zucchini and pepper and sauté over moderate heat for 3–4 minutes, until softened. Stir in the tomatoes, with salt and pepper to taste, and cook gently for 5 minutes.

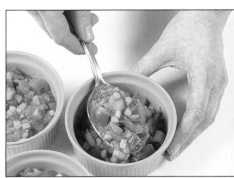

3 Divide the ratatouille among four individual ovenproof dishes or large ramekins, each with a capacity of about 1¼ cups.

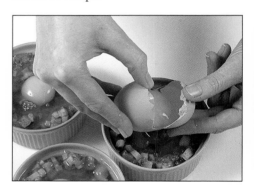

4 Make a small hollow in the center of each and break in an egg.

5 Grind some black pepper over the top of each cocotte and sprinkle with the Parmesan cheese. Bake for 10–15 minutes until the eggs are set. Sprinkle with the fresh parsley and serve at once.

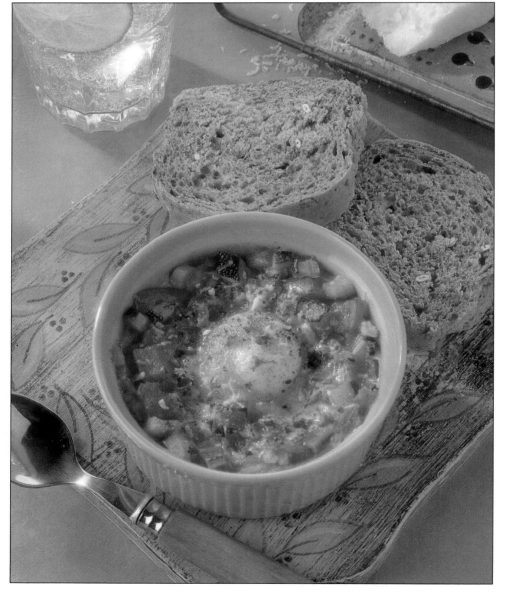

NUTRITIONAL NOTES	
Per Serving	
Energy	150 calories
Fat	10g
Saturated Fat	3g
Cholesterol	214.5mg

Mushroom and Fennel Hotpot

Marvellous flavors permeate this unusual vegetarian main course or accompaniment. Mushrooms provide useful amounts of vitamins, minerals and fiber.

INGREDIENTS

Serves 4

1 ounce dried shiitake mushrooms
1 small head of fennel or 4 celery stalks
2 tablespoons olive oil
12 shallots, peeled
2 cups button mushrooms, trimmed
    and halved
1¼ cups dry cider
1 ounce sun-dried tomatoes
2 tablespoons sun-dried tomato paste
1 bay leaf
chopped fresh parsley, to garnish

COOK'S TIP

Dried mushrooms swell up a great deal after soaking, so a little goes a long way both in terms of flavor and quantity.

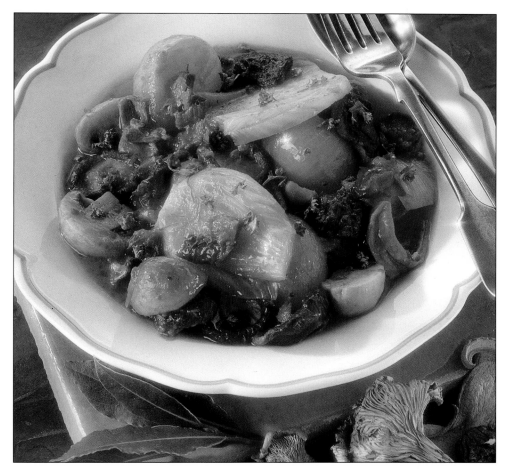

1 Place the dried mushrooms in a bowl. Pour over boiling water to cover and set aside for 10 minutes.

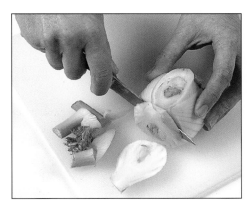

2 Coarsely chop the fennel or celery stalks and heat the oil in a flameproof casserole. Add the shallots and fennel or celery and sauté for about 10 minutes over moderate heat until the mixture is softened and lightly browned. Add the button mushrooms and fry for 2–3 minutes.

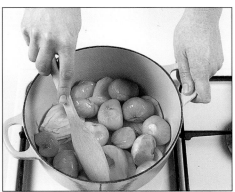

3 Drain the dried mushrooms, strain, and reserve the liquid. Cut up any large pieces and add to the pan.

NUTRITIONAL NOTES	
Per Serving	
Energy	170 calories
Fat	11.5g
Saturated Fat	1.5g
Cholesterol	0

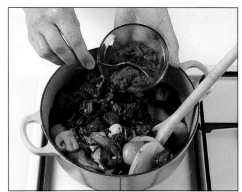

4 Pour in the cider and stir in the sun-dried tomatoes and the paste. Add the bay leaf. Bring to a boil, then lower the heat, cover the casserole and simmer gently for about 30 minutes.

5 If the mixture seems dry, stir in the reserved liquid from the soaked mushrooms. Reheat briefly, then remove the bay leaf and serve, sprinkled with plenty of chopped parsley.

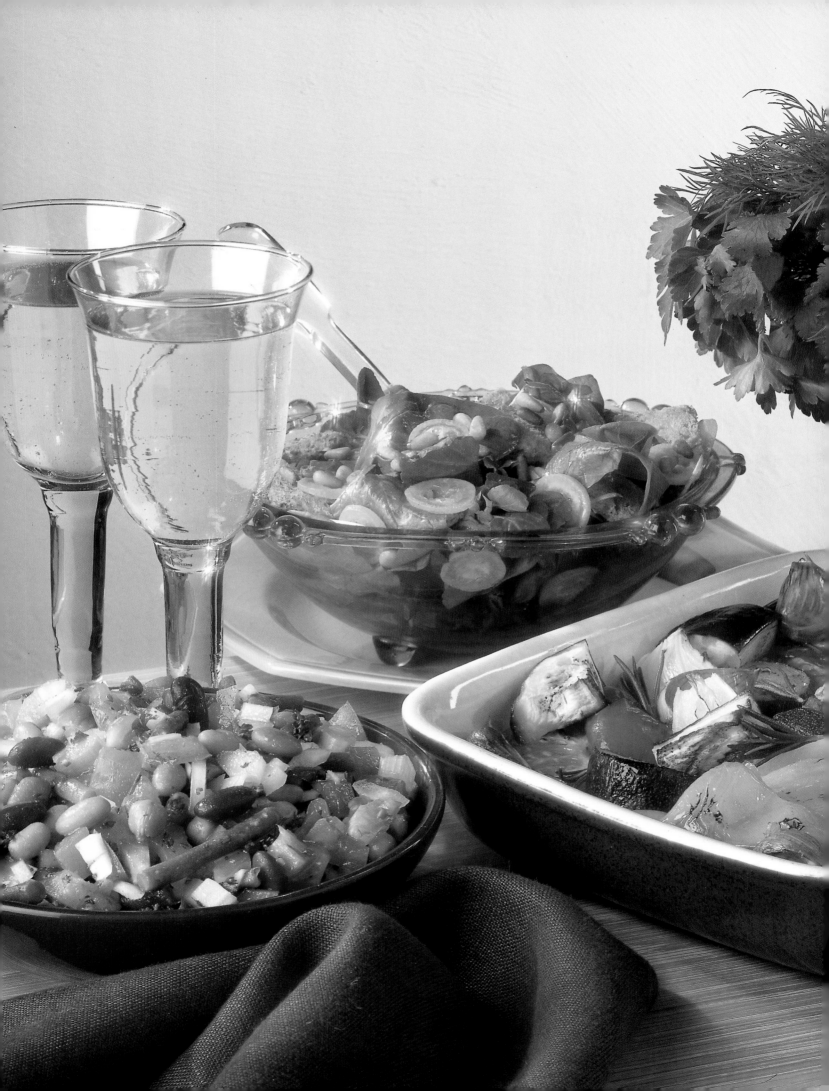

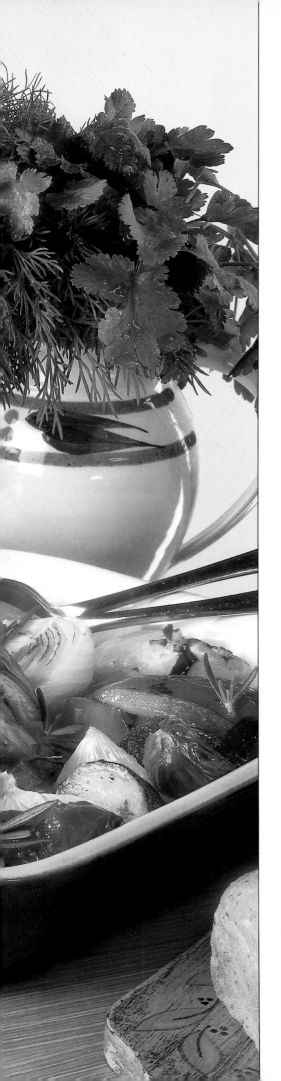

Salads and Vegetable Accompaniments

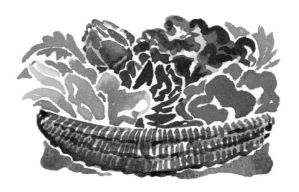

This chapter includes delicious accompaniments, based on the healthy starchy carbohydrate foods like rice, pasta, beans, lentils and potatoes, as well as recipes for interesting salads and cooked vegetable dishes. Fruit and vegetables provide valuable vitamins, minerals and fiber, essential for a high vitality diet. Your aim should be to include 5–6 portions daily (and this doesn't include potatoes). With such an amazing choice now readily available, this shouldn't be difficult. Shop wisely, buy fresh-looking produce, be adventurous to ensure a good variety and cook with care to preserve nutritional value. Make use of herbs, spices and garlic to tempt even the most fussy of vegetable eaters.

Bulgur Salad with Oranges and Almonds

Bulgur makes an excellent alternative to rice or pasta in this colorful salad.

INGREDIENTS

Serves 4
1 small green bell pepper
1 cup bulgur
2½ cups water
¼ cucumber, diced
½ cup chopped fresh mint
⅓ cup flaked almonds, toasted
grated rind and juice of 1 lemon
2 seedless oranges
salt and ground black pepper
mint sprigs, to garnish

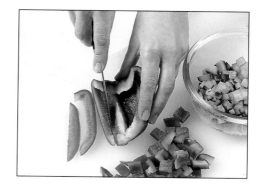

1 Using a sharp vegetable knife, carefully halve and seed the green pepper. Then cut it on a board into small cubes and put to one side.

2 Place the bulgur in a saucepan and add the water. Bring to a boil, lower the heat, cover and simmer for 10−15 minutes until tender. Alternatively, place the bulgur in a heatproof bowl, pour over boiling water and leave to soak for 30 minutes. Most, if not all, of the water should be absorbed; drain off any excess.

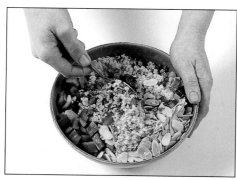

3 Toss the bulgur with the cucumber, green pepper, mint and toasted almonds in a serving bowl. Add the grated lemon rind and juice.

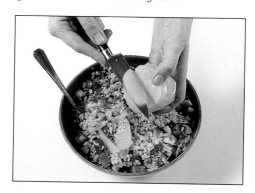

4 Cut the rind from the oranges, then, working over the bowl to catch the juice, cut the oranges into neat segments. Add to the bulgur mixture, then season and toss lightly. Garnish with the mint sprigs.

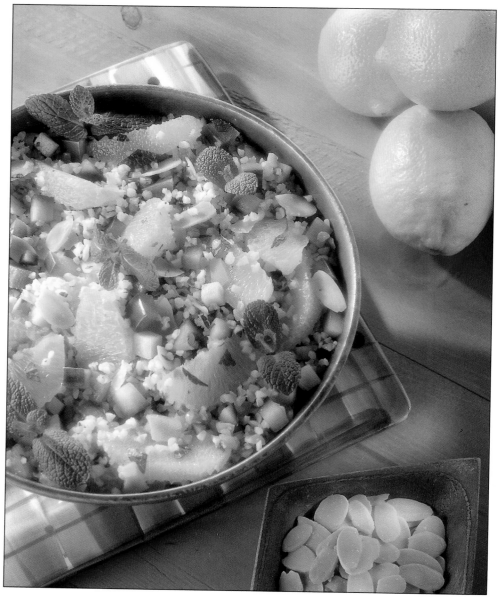

NUTRITIONAL NOTES	
Per Serving	
Energy	240 calories
Fat	6.5g
Saturated Fat	0.5g
Cholesterol	0

Fruited Brown Rice Salad

An oriental-style dressing gives this colorful rice salad extra piquancy. Whole grains like brown rice are unrefined, so they retain their natural fiber, vitamins and minerals.

INGREDIENTS

Serves 4–6

²/₃ cup brown rice
1 small red bell pepper, seeded and diced
7-ounce can corn kernels, drained
3 tablespoons golden raisins
8-ounce can pineapple pieces in fruit juice
2 tablespoons light soy sauce
1 tablespoon sunflower oil
1 tablespoon hazelnut oil
1 garlic clove, crushed
1 teaspoon finely chopped fresh ginger
salt and ground black pepper
4 scallions, sliced, to garnish

COOK'S TIP

Hazelnut oil gives a wonderfully distinctive flavor to any salad dressing. It is like olive oil, in that it contains mainly mono-unsaturated fats.

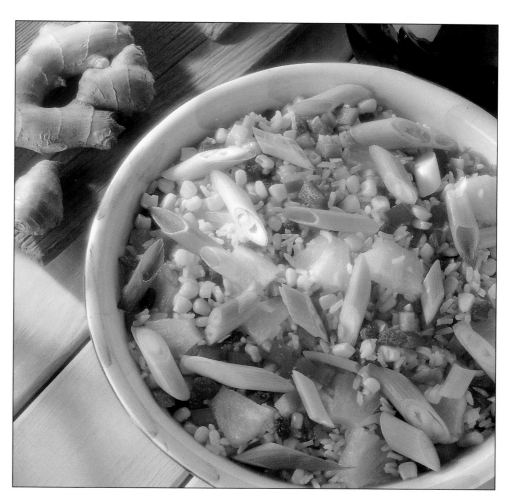

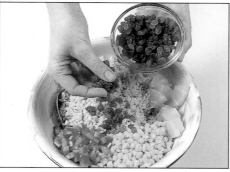

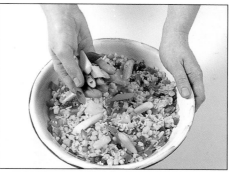

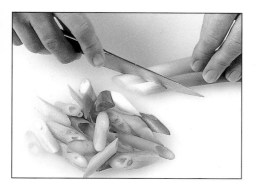

1 Cook the brown rice in a large saucepan of lightly salted boiling water for about 30 minutes, or until it is tender. Drain thoroughly and cool. Meanwhile, prepare the garnish by slicing the scallions at an angle and setting aside.

2 Turn the rice into a bowl and add the red pepper, corn and raisins. Drain the pineapple pieces, reserving the juice, then add them to the rice mixture and toss lightly.

3 Pour the reserved pineapple juice into a clean screw-top jar. Add the soy sauce, sunflower and hazelnut oils, garlic and ginger. Add some salt and pepper. Then close the jar tightly and shake well to combine.

4 Pour the dressing over the salad and toss well. Scatter the scallions over the top.

NUTRITIONAL NOTES
Per Serving

Energy	270 calories
Fat	7g
Saturated Fat	1g
Cholesterol	0

Cabbage Slaw with Date and Apple

Three types of cabbage are shredded together for serving raw, so that the maximum amount of vitamin C is retained in this cheerful salad.

INGREDIENTS

Serves 6–8
¼ small white cabbage, shredded
¼ small red cabbage, shredded
¼ small Savoy cabbage, shredded
1 cup dried pitted dates
3 eating apples
juice of 1 lemon
2 teaspoons caraway seeds

For the dressing
4 tablespoons olive oil
1 tablespoon cider vinegar
1 teaspoon honey
salt and ground black pepper

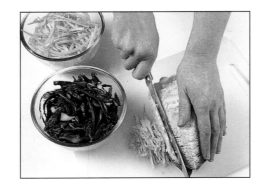

1 Finely shred all the cabbages and place them in a large salad bowl.

2 Chop the dates and add them to the cabbage.

3 Core the eating apples and slice them thinly into a mixing bowl. Add the lemon juice and toss together to prevent discoloration before adding to the salad bowl.

4 Make the dressing. Combine the oil, vinegar and honey in a screw-top jar. Add salt and pepper, then close the jar tightly and shake well. Pour the dressing over the salad, toss lightly, then sprinkle with the caraway seeds and toss again.

NUTRITIONAL NOTES
Per Serving

Energy	200 calories
Fat	8g
Saturated Fat	1g
Cholesterol	0

COOK'S TIP

Support your local orchards by looking out for different homegrown apples.

Sprouted Seed Salad

If you sprout beans, lentils and whole grains, it increases their nutritional value, and they make a deliciously crunchy salad.

INGREDIENTS

Serves 4
2 eating apples
4 ounces alfalfa sprouts
4 ounces bean sprouts
4 ounces aduki bean sprouts
¼ cucumber, sliced
2 bunches watercress, trimmed
1 cup salad cress

For the dressing
⅔ cup low-fat plain yogurt
juice of ½ lemon
bunch of chives, chopped
2 tablespoons chopped fresh herbs
ground black pepper

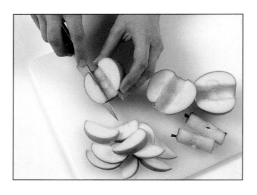

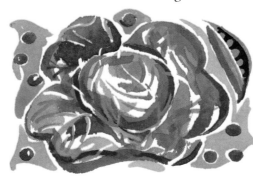

1 Core and slice the apples and mix with the other salad ingredients.

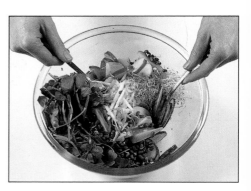

2 Mix the dressing ingredients in a measuring cup. Drizzle over the salad and toss together just before serving.

NUTRITIONAL NOTES
Per Serving

Energy	85 calories
Fat	1.5g
Saturated Fat	0.5g
Cholesterol	1.5mg

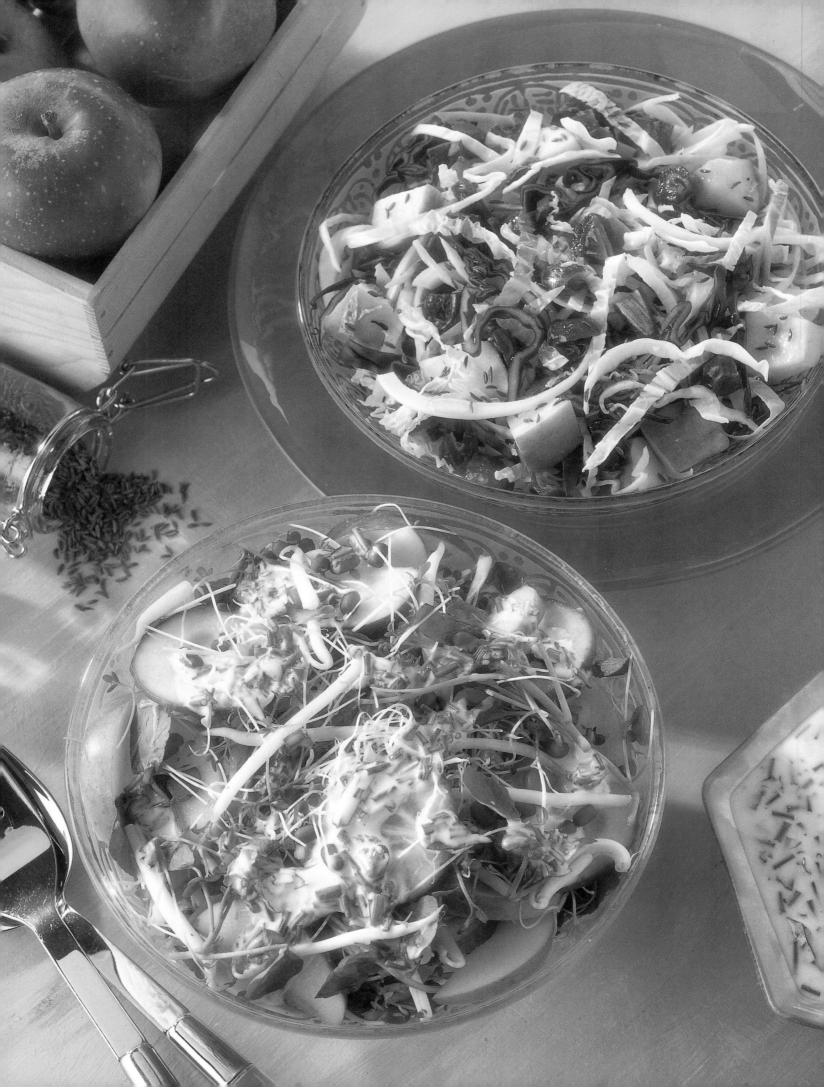

Citrus Green Leaf Salad with Croûtons

Whole wheat croûtons add a delicious crunch to leaf salads. The kumquats or orange segments provide a color contrast as well as a good helping of vitamin C.

INGREDIENTS

Serves 4–6

4 kumquats or 2 seedless oranges
7 ounces mixed green salad leaves
4 slices of whole wheat bread, crusts removed
2–3 tablespoons pine nuts, lightly toasted

For the dressing

grated rind of 1 lemon and 1 tablespoon juice
3 tablespoons olive oil
1 teaspoon whole-grain mustard
1 garlic clove, crushed

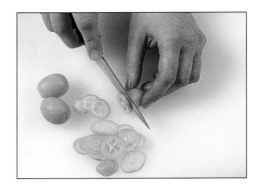

1 Thinly slice the kumquats, or peel and segment the oranges.

NUTRITIONAL NOTES	
Per Serving for 4	
Energy	250 calories
Fat	15g
Saturated fat	2g
Cholesterol	0

2 Tear all the salad leaves into bite-size pieces and place together in a large salad bowl.

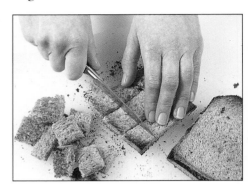

3 Toast the bread on both sides and cut into cubes. Add to the salad leaves with the sliced kumquats or orange segments.

4 Shake all the dressing ingredients together in a screw-top jar. Pour over the salad just before serving and sprinkle the pine nuts over the top.

Mixed Bean Salad with Tomato Dressing

All beans are a good source of vegetable protein, and minerals.

INGREDIENTS

Serves 4

4 ounces green beans
15-ounce can mixed beans, drained and rinsed
2 celery stalks, finely chopped
1 small onion, finely chopped
3 tomatoes, chopped
3 tablespoons chopped fresh parsley, to garnish

For the dressing

3 tablespoons olive oil
2 teaspoons red wine vinegar
1 garlic clove, crushed
1 tablespoon tomato chutney
salt and ground black pepper

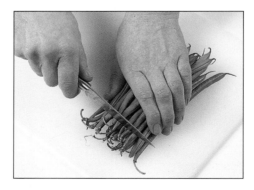

1 Remove the ends from the green beans, then cook the beans in boiling water for 5–6 minutes (or steam for 10 minutes) until tender. Drain, then refresh under cold running water and cut into thirds.

2 Place the green beans and canned beans in a bowl. Add the celery, onion and tomatoes and toss lightly.

3 Shake the dressing ingredients together in a jar. Pour over the salad and sprinkle with the parsley.

COOK'S TIP

Cans of mixed beans include several different types such as chick-peas, pinto, black-eye, red kidney, soy and aduki beans, and save the hassle of long soaking and cooking which dried beans require.

NUTRITIONAL NOTES	
Per Serving	
Energy	175 calories
Fat	9.5g
Saturated Fat	1.5g
Cholesterol	0

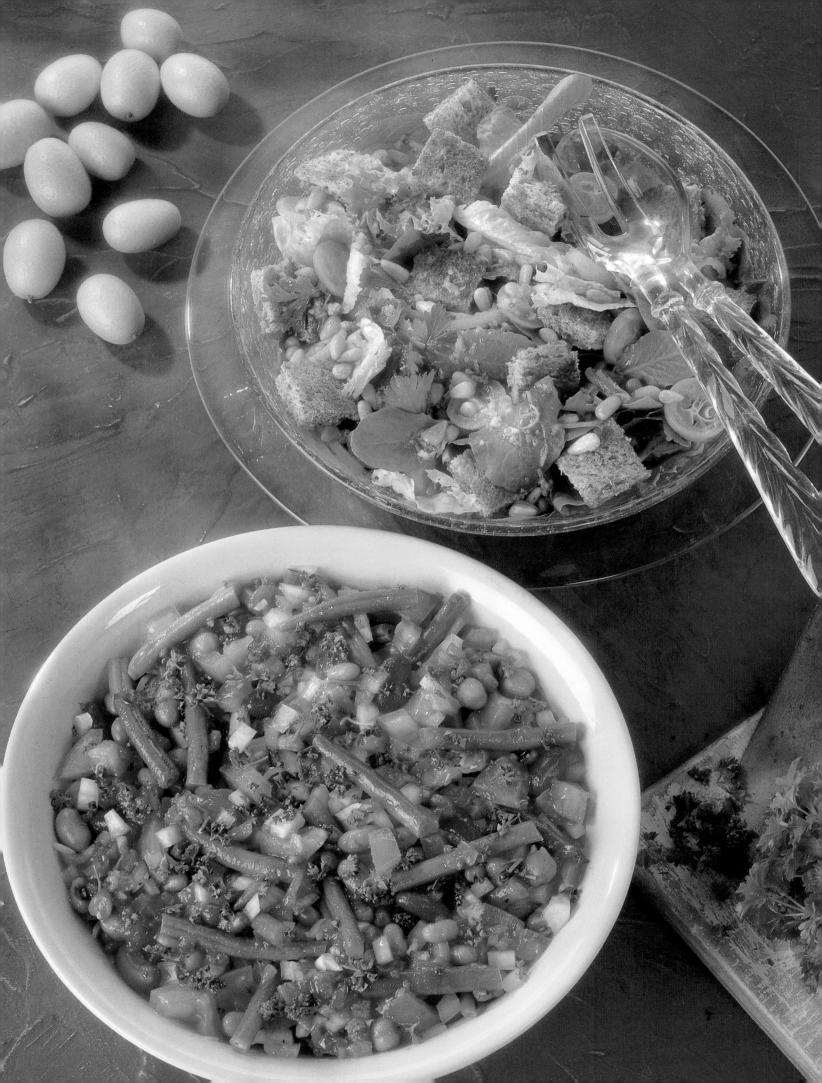

Baked Portobello Mushrooms

Portobello mushrooms, rich in B-group vitamins, have a wonderful flavor and are perfect for this nutty stuffing.

INGREDIENTS

Serves 4

2 tablespoons sunflower oil
8 Portobello mushrooms, wiped
1 onion, chopped
1 garlic clove, crushed
¼ cup rolled oats
8-ounce can chopped tomatoes
   with herbs
½ teaspoon hot pepper sauce
¼ cup pine nuts
¼ cup freshly grated Parmesan
   cheese
salt and ground black pepper

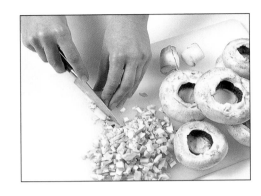

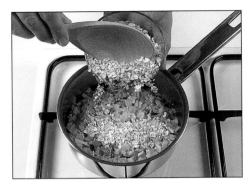

1 Preheat the oven to 375°F. Use a little of the oil to grease a shallow ovenproof dish lightly. The dish should be large enough to hold the mushroom caps in a single layer. Remove the mushroom stalks, chop them coarsely and set them aside. Reserve the whole mushroom caps.

2 Heat the oil in a small saucepan and sauté the onion, garlic and mushroom stalks until softened and lightly browned. Stir in the oats and cook for 1 minute more.

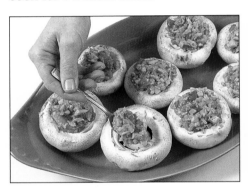

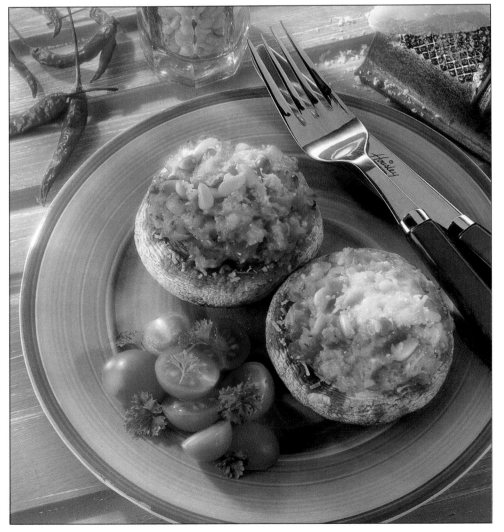

3 Stir in the tomatoes and hot pepper sauce and add salt and pepper to taste. Arrange the mushroom caps, gills uppermost, in the prepared dish. Divide the stuffing mixture among them.

4 Sprinkle the pine nuts and Parmesan cheese over the stuffed mushrooms. Bake for 25 minutes, until the mushrooms are tender and the topping is golden brown.

NUTRITIONAL NOTES	
Per Serving	
Energy	190 calories
Fat	13.5g
Saturated Fat	3g
Cholesterol	6.5mg

Roasted Mediterranean Vegetables

For a really colorful dish, try these vegetables roasted in olive oil with garlic and rosemary. The flavor is wonderfully intense.

INGREDIENTS

Serves 4

1 each red and yellow bell pepper
2 Spanish onions
2 large zucchini
1 large eggplant or 4 baby eggplant, trimmed
1 fennel bulb, thickly sliced
2 beefsteak tomatoes
8 fat garlic cloves
2 tablespoons olive oil
fresh rosemary sprigs
ground black pepper
lemon wedges and black olives, to garnish

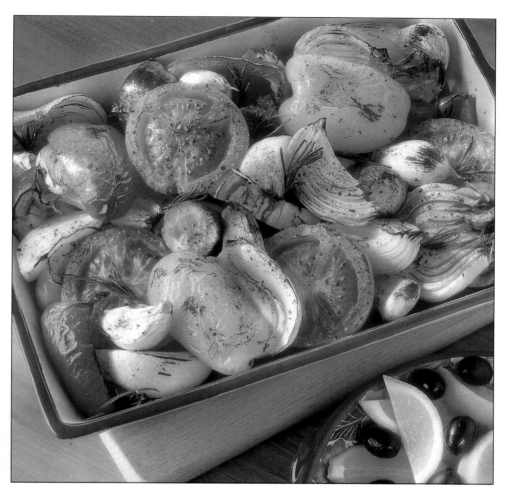

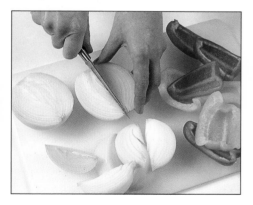

1 Halve and seed the peppers, then cut them into large chunks. Peel the onions and cut into thick wedges.

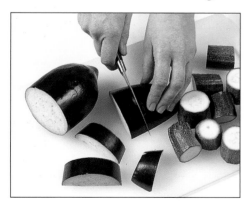

2 Cut the zucchini and eggplant into large chunks.

3 Preheat the oven to 425°F. Spread the peppers, onions, zucchini, eggplant and fennel in a lightly oiled, shallow ovenproof dish or roasting pan, or, if liked, arrange in rows to make a colorful design.

4 Cut each tomato in half and place, cut-side up, with the vegetables.

5 Tuck the garlic cloves among the vegetables, then brush them with the olive oil. Place some sprigs of rosemary among the vegetables and grind over some black pepper, particularly on the tomatoes.

6 Roast for 20–25 minutes, turning the vegetables halfway through the cooking time. Serve from the dish or on a flat platter, garnished with lemon wedges. Scatter some black olives over the top.

NUTRITIONAL NOTES	
Per Serving	
Energy	180 calories
Fat	8g
Saturated Fat	1g
Cholesterol	0

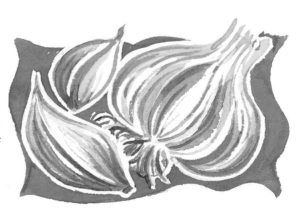

Mixed Vegetables with Aromatic Seeds

A healthy diet should include plenty of vegetables to provide fiber as well as vitamins and minerals. Here, spices transform everyday vegetables.

INGREDIENTS

Serves 4 – 6
1½ pounds small new potatoes
1 small cauliflower
6 ounces green beans
4 ounces frozen peas
small piece of fresh ginger
2 tablespoons sunflower oil
2 tablespoons cumin seeds
2 tablespoons black mustard seeds
2 tablespoons sesame seeds
juice of 1 lemon
ground black pepper
cilantro, to garnish (optional)

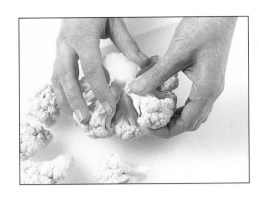

1 Scrub the potatoes, cut the cauliflower into small florets, and trim and halve the green beans.

2 Cook the vegetables in separate pans of lightly salted boiling water until tender, allowing 15–20 minutes for the potatoes, 8–10 minutes for the cauliflower and 4–5 minutes for the beans and peas. Drain thoroughly.

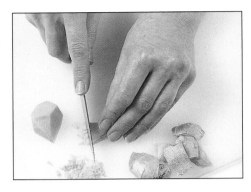

3 Using a small, sharp knife, peel and finely chop the fresh ginger.

4 Heat the oil. Add the ginger and seeds. Fry until they start to pop.

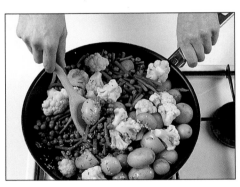

5 Add the vegetables and stir-fry for 2–3 minutes. Sprinkle over the lemon juice and season with pepper. Garnish with cilantro, if using.

COOK'S TIP

Other vegetables could be used, such as zucchini, leeks or broccoli. Buy whatever looks freshest and do not store vegetables for long periods as their vitamin content will deteriorate.

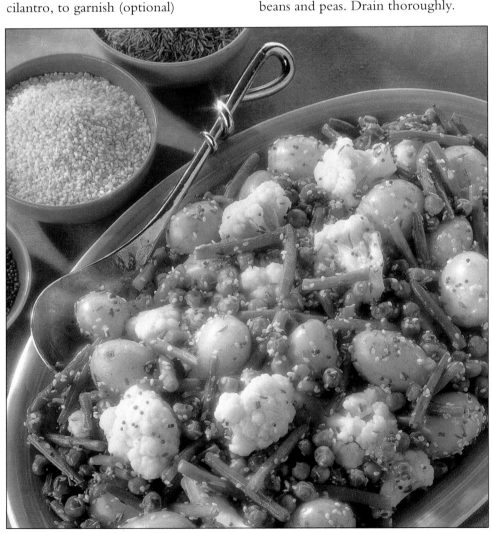

NUTRITIONAL NOTES
Per Serving for 4

Energy	285 calories
Fat	12.5g
Saturated Fat	1.5g
Cholesterol	0

Root Vegetable Casserole

Potatoes, carrots and parsnips are all complex carbohydrates and make a hearty, sustaining vegetable dish, high in fiber and vitamin C. The carrots are also an excellent source of beta-carotene, which is converted to vitamin A in the body.

INGREDIENTS

Serves 4–6
8 ounces carrots
8 ounces parsnips
1 tablespoon sunflower oil
pat of butter
1 tablespoon raw or brown sugar
1 pound baby new potatoes, scrubbed
8 ounces small onions, peeled
1²/₃ cups vegetable stock
1 tablespoon Worcestershire sauce
1 tablespoon tomato paste
1 teaspoon whole-grain mustard
2 bay leaves
salt and ground black pepper
chopped parsley, to garnish

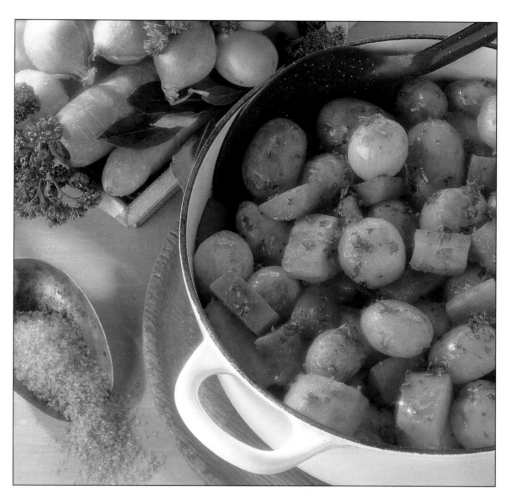

----- COOK'S TIP -----

Other vegetables could be added, such as leeks, mushrooms, sweet potato or celery. When they are in season, shelled chestnuts make a delicious addition.

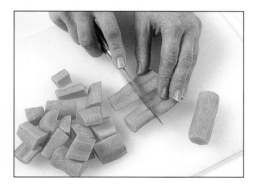

1 Peel the carrots and parsnips, then cut into large chunks.

2 Heat the oil, butter and sugar in a pan. Stir until the sugar dissolves.

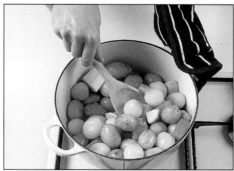

3 Add the potatoes, onions, carrots and parsnips. Sauté for 10 minutes, until the vegetables look glazed.

NUTRITIONAL NOTES	
Per Serving for 4	
Energy	215 calories
Fat	5.5g
Saturated Fat	1g
Cholesterol	3mg

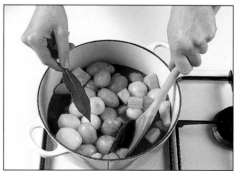

4 Mix the vegetable stock, Worcestershire sauce, tomato paste and mustard in a pitcher. Stir well, then pour over the vegetables. Add the bay leaves. Bring to a boil, then lower the heat, cover and cook gently for about 30 minutes, until the vegetables are tender.

5 Remove the bay leaves, add salt and pepper to taste and serve, sprinkled with the parsley.

Concertina Garlic Potatoes

With a low-fat topping these make a superb meal in themselves, or enjoy them as a nutritious accompaniment.

INGREDIENTS

Serves 4

4 large baking potatoes
2 garlic cloves, cut into slivers
4 tablespoons fat-free sour cream
4 tablespoons low-fat plain yogurt
2 tablespoons chopped chives
6–8 watercress sprigs, finely chopped (optional)

NUTRITIONAL NOTES	
Per Serving	
Energy	195 calories
Fat	3.5g
Saturated Fat	2g
Cholesterol	10mg

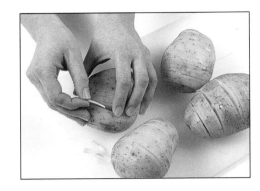

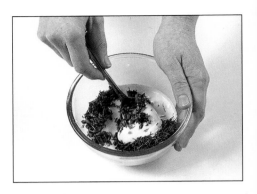

1 Preheat the oven to 400°F. Slice each potato at ¼-inch intervals, cutting almost to the base, so that they retain their shape. Slip the garlic between some of the cuts.

—— COOK'S TIP ——

The most suitable potatoes for baking are of the floury variety. The best, of course, are Idaho, but you may find local varieties just as good; often labeled simply "baking."

2 Place the garlic-filled potatoes in a roasting pan and bake for 1–1¼ hours or until soft when tested with a knife. Meanwhile, mix the sour cream and low-fat yogurt in a bowl. Then stir in the chopped chives, along with the watercress, if using.

3 Serve the baked potatoes on individual plates, with a dollop of the yogurt and cream mixture on top of each.

Potato, Leek and Tomato Bake

INGREDIENTS

Serves 4

1½ pounds potatoes
2 leeks, trimmed and sliced
3 large tomatoes, sliced
a few fresh rosemary sprigs, crushed
1 garlic clove, crushed
1¼ cups vegetable stock
1 tablespoon olive oil
salt and ground black pepper

NUTRITIONAL NOTES	
Per Serving	
Energy	180 calories
Fat	3.5g
Saturated Fat	0.5g
Cholesterol	0

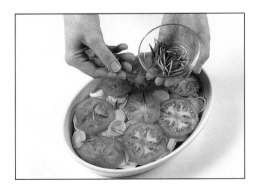

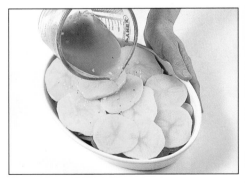

1 Preheat the oven to 350°F and grease a 5-cup shallow ovenproof casserole. Scrub and thinly slice the potatoes. Then layer them with the leeks and tomatoes in the dish, sprinkling some crushed rosemary between the layers and ending with a layer of potatoes.

2 Add the garlic to the stock, stir in salt and pepper to taste and pour over the vegetables. Brush the top layer of potatoes with the olive oil.

3 Bake for 1¼–1½ hours or until the potatoes are tender and the topping is golden and slightly crisp.

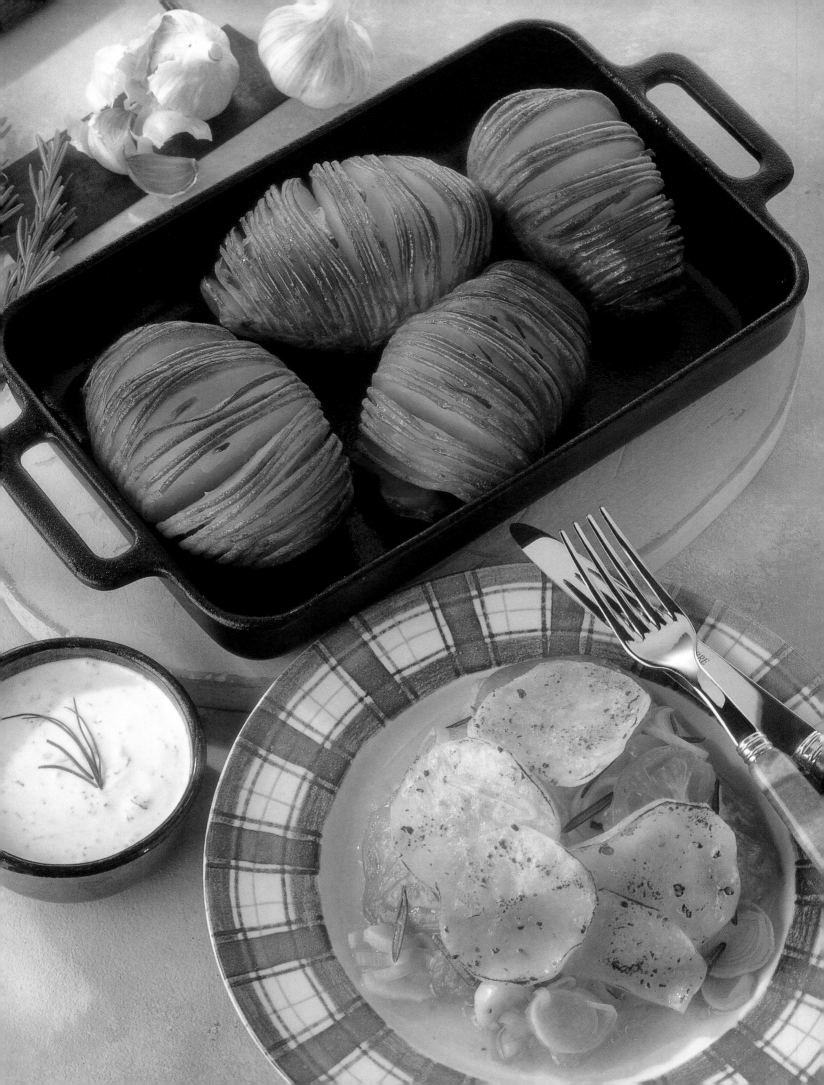

Tomato, Pistachio and Sesame Pilaf

INGREDIENTS

Serves 4

3 tomatoes
1 red bell pepper
1⅓ cups brown basmati rice
2½ cups vegetable stock or water
pinch of saffron strands soaked in
   1 tablespoon boiling water
pinch of salt
4–5 cardamom pods
¼ cup pistachio nuts, coarsely chopped
2 tablespoons sesame seeds, toasted

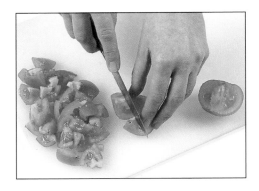

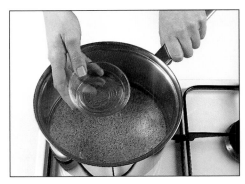

1 Place the tomatoes in boiling water for 30 seconds to loosen the skins, then peel and chop.

2 Using a sharp knife, halve, seed and chop the red pepper.

3 Wash the rice in a strainer under cold running water, then turn into a saucepan. Add the stock or water, soaked saffron liquid and salt. Bring to the boil, then lower the heat, cover and simmer for 25 minutes.

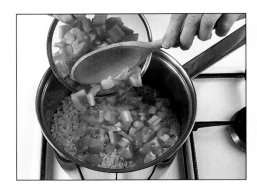

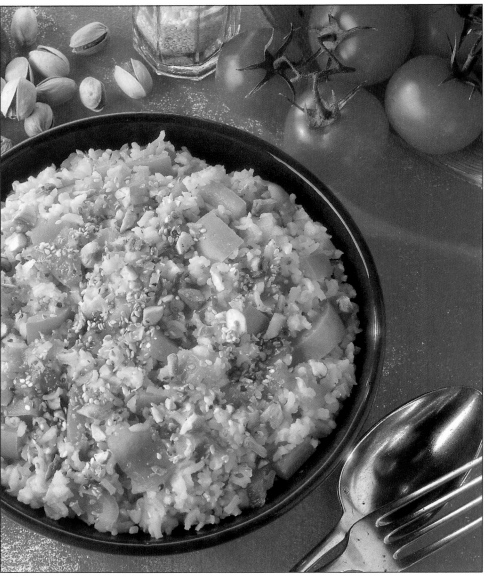

4 Add the tomatoes and peppers to the rice. Crush the cardamom pods, extract the seeds and stir them into the mixture. Cook for another 5–10 minutes, until the rice is tender and all the liquid has been absorbed. If the liquid is absorbed before the rice is cooked, add a little more. It should not be necessary to drain the rice.

5 Turn the rice into a serving dish and sprinkle the pistachio nuts and sesame seeds over the top.

NUTRITIONAL NOTES	
Per Serving	
Energy	315 calories
Fat	10g
Saturated Fat	1.5g
Cholesterol	0

Winter Vegetable Stir-fry

Brussels sprouts are not always popular, but taste absolutely delicious when steamed and swiftly stir-fried. As a bonus, more of their vitamin B and C content is preserved.

INGREDIENTS

Serves 4

12 ounces Brussels sprouts
2 zucchini
1 tablespoon sunflower or nut oil
12 shallots, peeled
1 garlic clove, crushed
small piece of fresh ginger, peeled and
    finely chopped
¼ cup walnut pieces

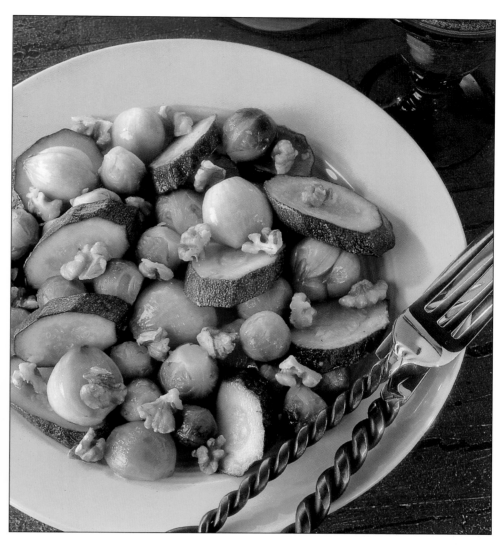

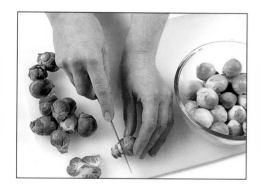

1 If necessary, trim the sprouts and remove any dirty outside leaves.

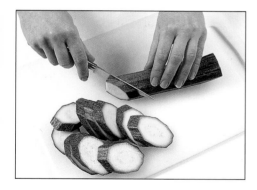

2 Cut the zucchini into even-size diagonal slices.

3 Steam the Brussels sprouts for about 7–10 minutes, or until they are just tender. Drain, if necessary, and set aside.

4 Heat the oil in a frying pan or wok. Add the shallots and zucchini and stir-fry for 2–3 minutes.

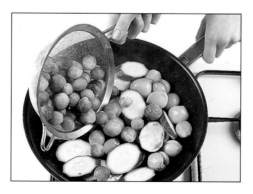

5 Add the sprouts, garlic and ginger and stir-fry for 2 minutes more. Sprinkle over the walnut pieces, toss them with the vegetable mixture and serve immediately.

COOK'S TIP

Choose small, tight Brussels sprouts which don't need to be trimmed or have their outside leaves removed. The darker outside leaves are rich in vitamins and minerals. Shredded cabbage could be used instead of Brussels sprouts, and chestnuts in place of walnuts. Vacuum-packed chestnuts are cooked and ready to use.

NUTRITIONAL NOTES
Per Serving

Energy	125 calories
Fat	8.5g
Saturated Fat	1g
Cholesterol	0

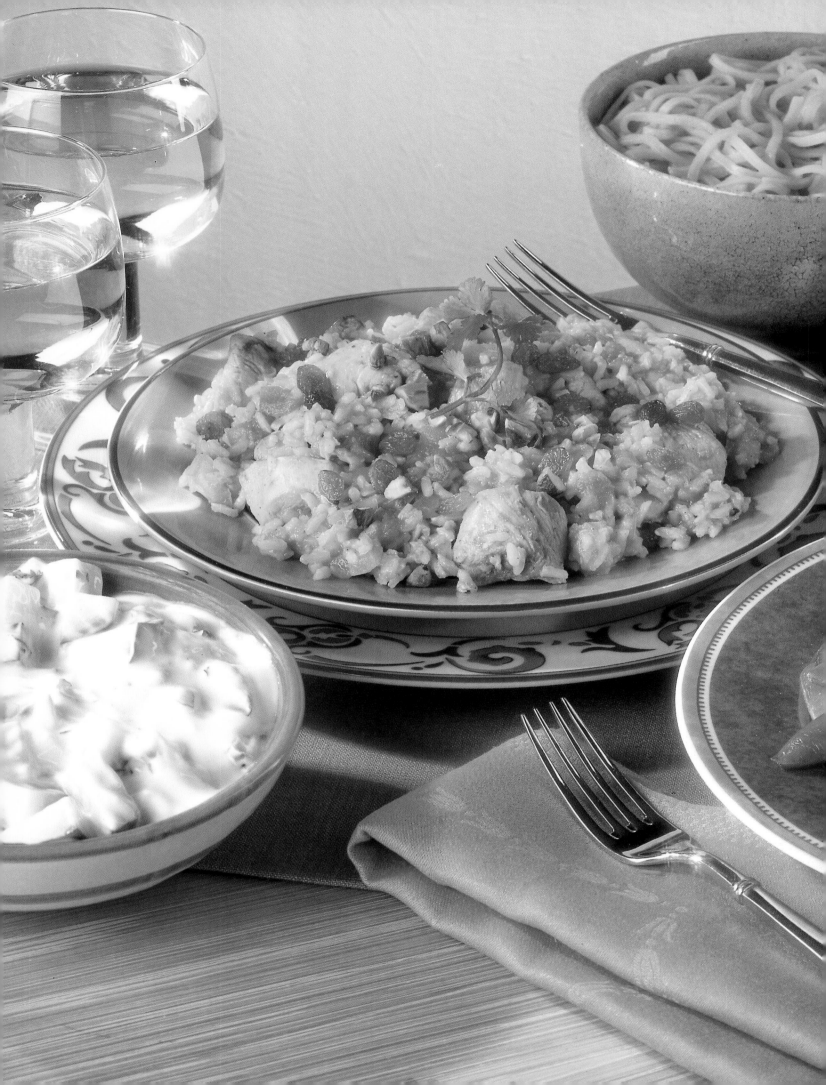

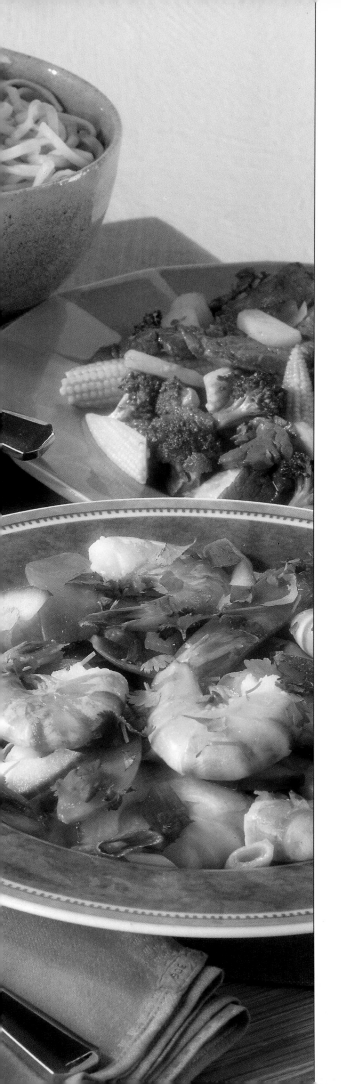

MAIN MEALS

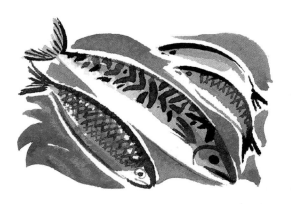

This chapter contains tempting ideas for meat, poultry, fish and vegetarian meals. The main meal of the day is likely to provide a considerable amount of your daily energy intake, so be sure you're getting good nutritional value for your calories. The meat recipes use lean cuts, and vegetables, dried fruits, beans and lentils are incorporated into the dishes to increase fiber, reduce fat and build in extra vitamins and minerals. Whether cooking for simple midweek meals or special occasions, there's plenty to whet the appetite.

Beef and Broccoli Stir-fry with Black Bean Sauce

INGREDIENTS

Serves 4

1 tablespoon sunflower oil
8 ounces tenderloin or round steak, thinly sliced across the grain
8 ounces broccoli
4-ounce can baby corn, diagonally halved
3 – 4 tablespoons water
2 leeks, diagonally sliced
8-ounce can water chestnuts, drained and sliced

For the marinade

1 tablespoon fermented black beans
2 tablespoons dark soy sauce
2 tablespoons cider vinegar
1 tablespoon sunflower oil
1 teaspoon sugar
2 garlic cloves, crushed
1-inch piece of fresh ginger, peeled and finely chopped

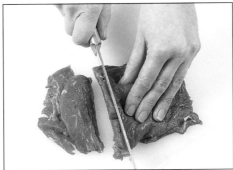

1 Make the marinade. Mash the fermented black beans in a non-metallic bowl. Stir in the remaining ingredients. Cut the steak into thin slices across the grain, then add them to the marinade.

2 Stir the steak well to coat it in the marinade. Cover the bowl and leave for several hours or overnight in the fridge.

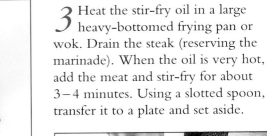

3 Heat the stir-fry oil in a large heavy-bottomed frying pan or wok. Drain the steak (reserving the marinade). When the oil is very hot, add the meat and stir-fry for about 3 – 4 minutes. Using a slotted spoon, transfer it to a plate and set aside.

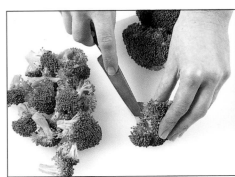

4 Cut the broccoli into small florets. Reheat the oil remaining in the pan, add the broccoli and corn and stir in the water. Cover and steam gently for 5 minutes, or until the vegetables are tender, but still have some "bite."

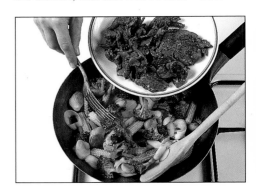

5 Add the leeks and water chestnuts to the broccoli mixture and toss over the heat for 1 – 2 minutes. Return the meat to the pan, pour over the reserved marinade and toss the mixture over a high heat.

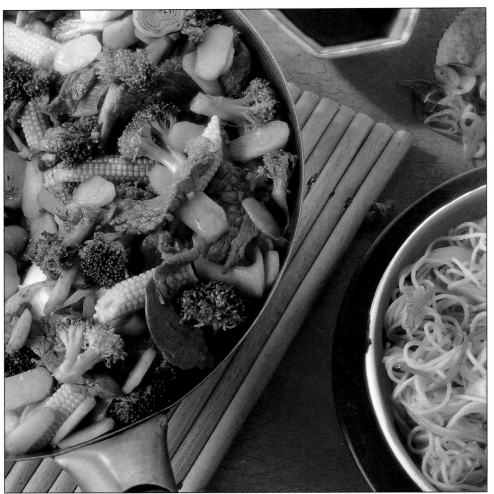

NUTRITIONAL NOTES	
Per Serving	
Energy	190 calories
Fat	9g
Saturated Fat	2g
Cholesterol	33.5mg

Beef and Lentil Pies

In this variation of shepherd's pie, lentils are substituted for some of the meat to produce a dish that is lower in fat and higher in fiber. Some red meat is included to boost the iron.

INGREDIENTS

Serves 4

1 cup green lentils
8 ounces extra-lean ground beef
1 onion, chopped
2 celery stalks, chopped
1 large carrot, chopped
1 garlic clove, crushed
15-ounce can chopped tomatoes
2 teaspoons brewer's yeast powder
1 bay leaf

For the topping

1 pound potatoes, peeled and cut into
　　large chunks
1 pound parsnips, peeled and cut into
　　large chunks
4 tablespoons low-fat plain yogurt
3 tablespoons chopped chives
4 teaspoons freshly grated
　　Parmesan cheese
2 tomatoes, sliced
1/4 cup pine nuts (optional)

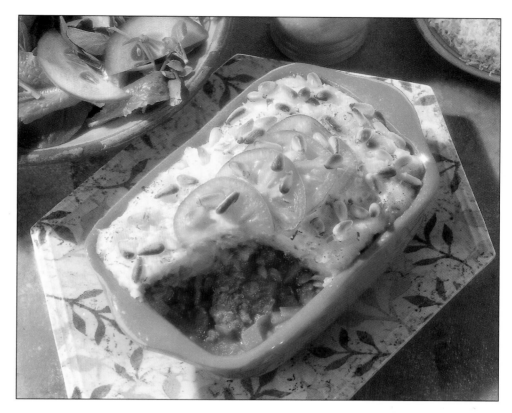

1 Place the lentils in a pan and pour in cold water to cover. Bring to a boil, then boil for 10 minutes.

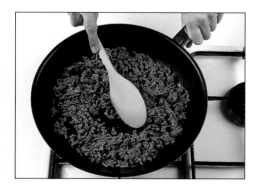

2 Meanwhile, brown the beef in a saucepan, without any extra fat. Stir in the onion, celery, carrot and garlic. Cook gently for 5 minutes, then stir in the tomatoes.

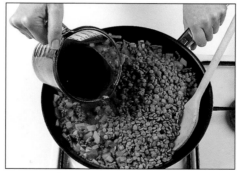

3 Drain the lentils, reserving 1¼ cups of the cooking water in a measuring cup. Add the lentils to the meat mixture, then dissolve the yeast in the cooking water and stir it in. Add the bay leaf, bring to a boil, then lower the heat, cover the pan and cook gently for 20 minutes.

4 Make the topping. Bring a saucepan of lightly salted water to a boil and cook the potatoes and parsnips for about 15 minutes, until tender. Drain, turn into a bowl, and mash with the yogurt and chives. Preheat the broiler.

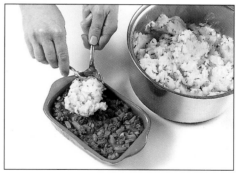

5 Remove the bay leaf and divide the mixture among four small dishes. Spoon over the potato mixture. Sprinkle with Parmesan and garnish with tomato slices. Sprinkle pine nuts over the top, if using, and broil the pies for a few minutes until the topping is crisp and golden.

NUTRITIONAL NOTES	
Per Portion	
Energy	470 calories
Fat	10.5g
Saturated Fat	2.5g
Cholesterol	36.5mg

Moroccan Lamb Tagine with Couscous

A tagine is a Moroccan stew that typically combines meat and fruit with aromatic herbs and spices. The result is a low-fat casserole with extra vitamins and fiber.

INGREDIENTS

Serves 4

1 tablespoon sunflower oil
12 ounces lean, boneless lamb, cubed
1 large onion, chopped
1 garlic clove, crushed
2½ cups stock
1 cinnamon stick
small piece of fresh ginger, peeled and finely chopped
1 teaspoon clear honey
grated rind and juice of 1 orange
1 eggplant
2–3 tablespoons salt
4 tomatoes, peeled and chopped
²⁄₃ cup dried apricots, halved
2 tablespoons chopped fresh cilantro
ground black pepper

For the couscous

1½ cups couscous
1²⁄₃ cups water
pinch of saffron strands, soaked in 1 tablespoon boiling water (optional)
pat of butter
1 teaspoon orange flower water (optional)

COOK'S TIP

Couscous is a cereal made from ground wheat (semolina) mixed with water and salt and shaped into tiny pellets. Like rice, it can either be served hot with meat, poultry or vegetable dishes, or cold, mixed with nuts and dried fruits for a tasty salad. If you buy packaged couscous, cook as directed on the package.

1 Heat the oil in a large saucepan or flameproof casserole. Add the lamb and onion and sauté for 5 minutes until lightly browned.

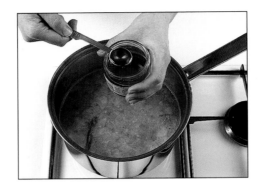

2 Add the garlic, then stir in the stock, cinnamon, ginger, honey, orange rind and juice. Bring to a boil, then lower the heat, cover the pan and simmer gently for 45 minutes.

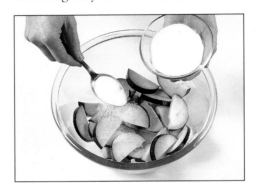

3 Meanwhile, wipe the eggplant and cut into pieces. Place the pieces in a mixing bowl. Sprinkle the eggplant with salt and leave for about 30 minutes so that the bitter juices are drawn out.

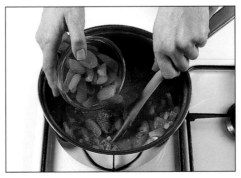

4 Add the chopped tomatoes and dried apricots to the casserole. Rinse the eggplant, then drain well and add to the tagine. Cover and cook for another 45 minutes or until the lamb is tender.

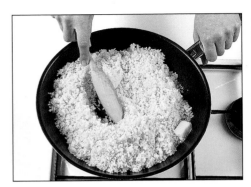

5 About 20 minutes before the lamb is ready, cook the couscous, either in a separate pan or in a steamer above the stew. Start by placing the couscous in a bowl, pour over lightly salted boiling water to cover and sprinkle with the infused saffron, if using. Soak for 5 minutes. Melt the butter in a saucepan, add the couscous and cook over moderate heat for 3–5 minutes. Alternatively, place the couscous in a steamer set above the stew and steam it for 6–7 minutes. Turn the couscous into a bowl and sprinkle with orange flower water, if using.

6 Stir the cilantro into the tagine just before serving with the couscous.

NUTRITIONAL NOTES	
Per Serving (with couscous)	
Energy	430 calories
Fat	14.5g
Saturated Fat	6g
Cholesterol	75mg

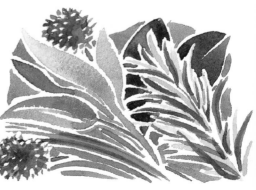

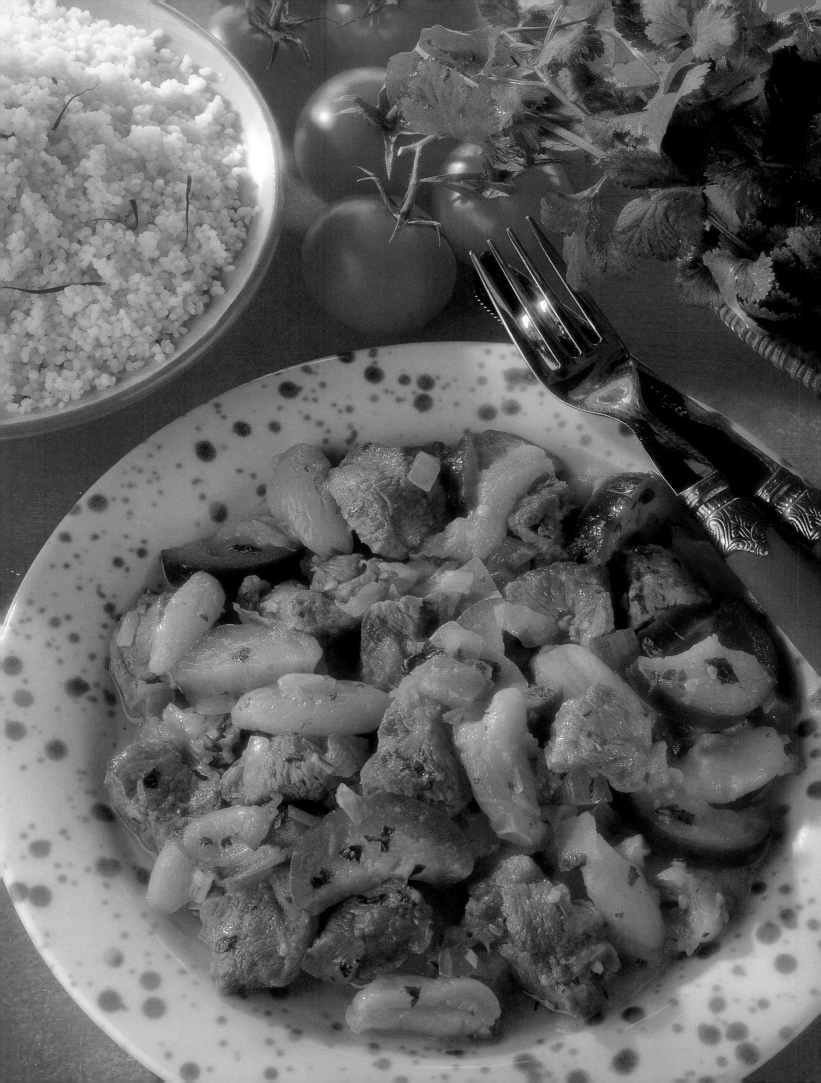

Chili Lamb and Potato Goulash

INGREDIENTS

Serves 4

1 pound lean lamb, cubed
1 onion, coarsely chopped
1 garlic clove, crushed
14-ounce can chopped tomatoes
1¼ cups stock
1 tablespoon tomato chutney
1 tablespoon paprika
2 green chilies, seeded and chopped
1 pound small new potatoes, scrubbed
1 red bell pepper, seeded
   and chopped
1 bunch fresh fenugreek leaves
   (optional)
5 ounces young spinach leaves
salt and ground black pepper

To serve

⅔ cup low-fat plain yogurt
paprika, for dusting
2 scallions, chopped

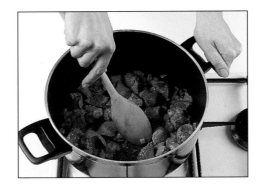

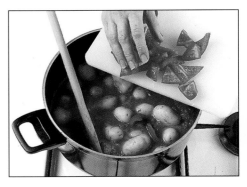

1 Place the lamb in a flameproof casserole over low heat until the fat runs, then raise the heat and fry until lightly browned. Drain off any excess fat, then add the onion and garlic and sauté for 3–4 minutes, until the onions are lightly browned. Add the tomatoes, stock, chutney, paprika and chilies to the casserole. Bring to a boil, then cover and cook gently for 1 hour.

2 Add the potatoes and pepper, replace the lid and cook for another 20–25 minutes, until the potatoes are tender. Add more stock, if necessary. Season to taste.

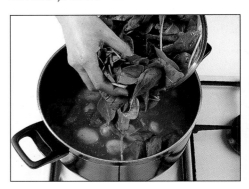

3 If using the fenugreek, bring a saucepan of water to the boil, add the bunch of leaves and blanch for 1 minute to remove any bitterness. Drain well and add to the casserole. Tear the spinach leaves into smaller pieces. Add them to the casserole and cook for 5 minutes – the spinach will wilt down rapidly, so don't worry about the large quantity when raw.

4 Serve in individual heated bowls. Spoon a little yogurt over each portion, dust with paprika and sprinkle over some chopped scallions.

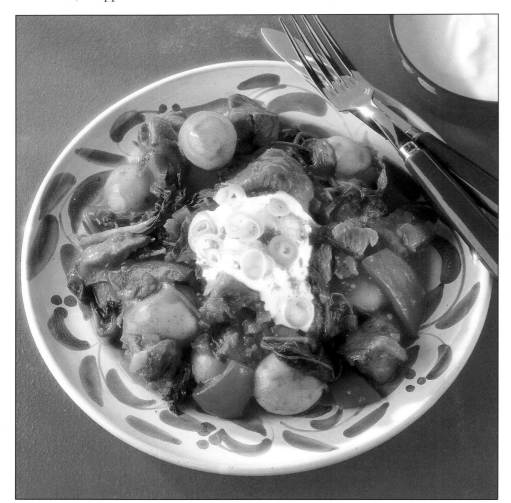

NUTRITIONAL NOTES	
Per Serving (without yogurt topping)	
Energy	335 calories
Fat	11.5g
Saturated Fat	5g
Cholesterol	89mg

Pork with Prunes

Prunes are an excellent source of fiber and beta-carotene. They also provide iron.

INGREDIENTS

Serves 4

1 cup prunes, pitted
1¼ cups dry white wine, cider or
  apple juice
1 tablespoon sunflower oil
4 lean pork cutlets
1 tablespoon red currant jelly
1 tablespoon cornstarch
¾ cup low-fat plain yogurt
salt and ground black pepper
sprigs of fresh parsley, to garnish
carrots and green vegetables, to serve
  (optional)

NUTRITIONAL NOTES	
Per Serving	
Energy	390 calories
Fat	12.5g
Saturated Fat	4g
Cholesterol	88mg

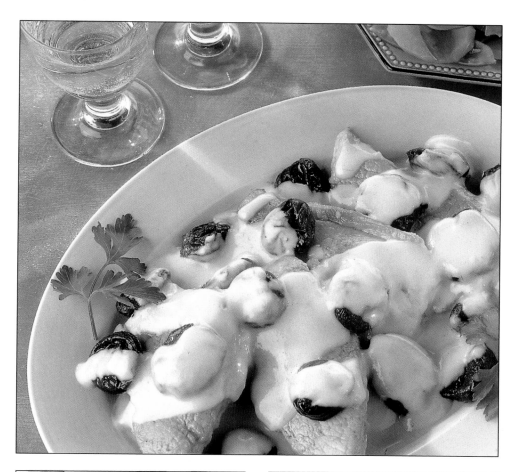

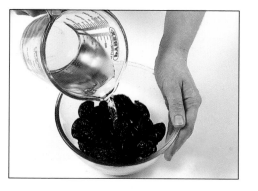

1 Place the prunes in a mixing bowl and pour over the white wine, cider or apple juice. Leave them to plump up while you cook the pork.

2 Trim the pork cutlets by removing any fat. Heat the sunflower oil in a large heavy-bottomed frying pan. Then add the pork and fry until browned on both sides. Drain off any excess fat.

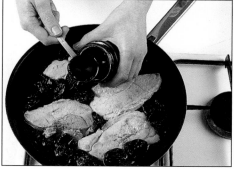

3 Pour in the prunes with the liquid, and add the red currant jelly. Season to taste. Bring to a boil, then lower the heat, cover the pan and simmer for about 20 minutes, until the pork is tender.

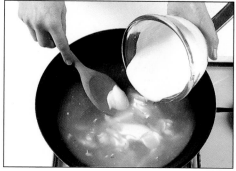

4 Stir the cornstarch and yogurt together in a bowl. Using a slotted spoon, transfer the pork and prunes to a warmed serving dish. Cover and keep hot. Gradually add the yogurt mixture to the liquid in the pan, stirring constantly over the heat until the sauce has thickened.

5 Pour the sauce over the pork and prunes and garnish with the parsley sprigs. Serve at once, with carrots and seasonal green vegetables, if you like.

Braised Venison with Orange and Cranberries

INGREDIENTS

Serves 4

1½ pounds venison
1 tablespoon olive oil
16 shallots, peeled
1 garlic clove, crushed
2½ cups stock
juice of 2 oranges
1 tablespoon orange marmalade
small piece of fresh ginger, peeled and
  finely chopped
1 teaspoon honey
few fresh thyme sprigs
4 large carrots, cut into thick chunks
1¼ cups fresh cranberries
2 cups button mushrooms
2 tablespoons chopped walnuts
salt and ground black pepper
fresh thyme sprigs and whole wheat
  toast croûtes, to garnish

1 Cut the venison into small pieces. Heat the oil in a flameproof casserole and sauté the venison with the whole shallots and the crushed garlic for 5 minutes, or until the shallots are lightly browned.

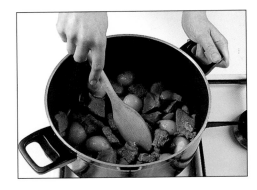

2 Add the stock, orange juice, marmalade, ginger and honey and stir well.

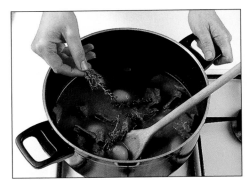

3 Add the sprigs of thyme and bring to a boil. Then lower the heat, cover the casserole with a lid and cook gently for 1½ hours.

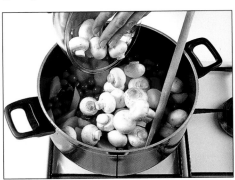

4 Add the carrots, cranberries and mushrooms to the casserole and cook gently for another 20–30 minutes, or until the venison is tender, adding a little extra stock if necessary.

5 Remove the thyme sprigs and add salt and pepper to taste. Sprinkle the chopped walnuts over the top and garnish with the fresh thyme sprigs and whole wheat toast croûtes.

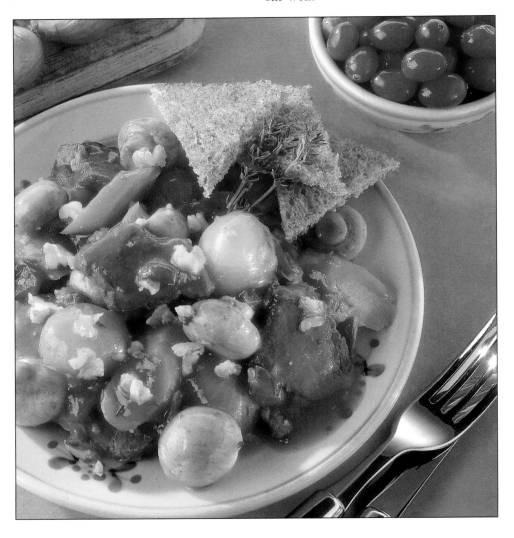

NUTRITIONAL NOTES	
Per Serving	
Energy	365 calories
Fat	11.5g
Saturated Fat	3g
Cholesterol	143.5mg

Turkey Picadillo

Using ground turkey rather than beef for this Mexican-style dish makes it much lower in fat. Serve as a filling for soft wheat tortillas and then top with some low-fat plain yogurt for a tasty meal. Alternatively, serve the Picadillo as a topping for baked potatoes.

INGREDIENTS

Serves 4

1 tablespoon sunflower oil
1 onion, chopped
1 pound ground turkey
1−2 garlic cloves, crushed
1 green chili, seeded and
    finely chopped
6 tomatoes, peeled and chopped
1 tablespoon tomato paste or sun-dried
    tomato paste
½ teaspoon ground cumin
1 yellow or orange bell pepper, seeded
    and chopped
⅓ cup raisins
½ cup flaked almonds, toasted
3 tablespoons chopped cilantro
⅔ cup low-fat plain yogurt
2−3 scallions, finely chopped
4 soft tortillas
salt and ground black pepper
shredded lettuce, to serve

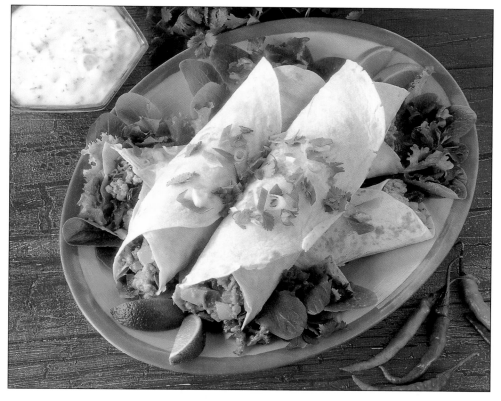

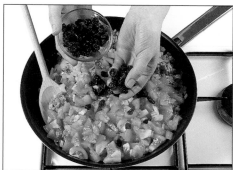

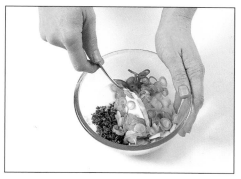

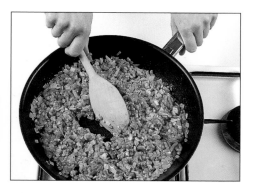

1 Heat the oil in a large frying pan and add the chopped onion. Cook gently for 5 minutes, until soft. Then stir in the ground turkey and garlic and cook gently for another 5 minutes.

2 Stir in the chili, tomatoes, tomato paste, cumin, yellow or orange pepper and raisins. Cover and cook over gentle heat for 15 minutes, stirring occasionally and adding a little water if necessary.

3 Stir in the toasted almonds, with about two-thirds of the chopped cilantro. Add salt and freshly ground black pepper to taste.

4 Turn the yogurt into a bowl. Stir in the remaining cilantro and the scallions.

5 Heat the tortillas in a dry frying pan, without oil, for 15−20 seconds. Place some shredded lettuce and turkey mixture on each tortilla, roll up like a pancake and transfer to a plate. Top with a generous spoonful of the low-fat yogurt and cilantro mixture and serve immediately.

NUTRITIONAL NOTES	
Per Serving	
Energy	460 calories
Fat	12.5g
Saturated Fat	2g
Cholesterol	57mg

Chicken Biryani

A wonderfully spicy baked Indian dish made with brown basmati rice.

INGREDIENTS

Serves 6

2 tablespoons sunflower oil
1 large onion, chopped
2 garlic cloves, crushed
small piece of fresh ginger, peeled and finely chopped
1½ pounds boned chicken breasts or thighs, skinned and cubed
6 cardamom pods
2 teaspoons ground cumin
2 teaspoons ground coriander
½ teaspoon cayenne pepper
6 cloves
1 cinnamon stick
½ teaspoon whole black peppercorns
2 bay leaves
juice of 1 lemon
4 large tomatoes, peeled and chopped
²/₃ cup chicken stock
few drops of rosewater (optional)
low-fat plain yogurt or raita, to serve

For the rice
1²/₃ cups brown basmati rice
2 tablespoons warm milk
pinch of saffron strands
1 tablespoon sunflower oil
1 small onion, thinly sliced
3 cups chicken stock
few drops of rosewater (optional)

For the garnish
coarsely chopped pistachio nuts
golden raisins
cilantro sprigs

COOK'S TIP

A minty potato raita is marvelously cooling with the biryani. Spoon ⅔ cup low-fat plain yogurt into a bowl. Stir in 1 teaspoon mint sauce, then add 8 ounces cooked, cubed potato. Mix gently and sprinkle with a little cayenne pepper before serving.

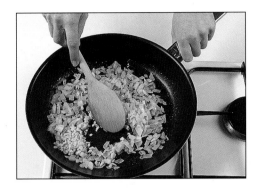

1 Preheat the oven to 325°F. Heat the oil in a frying pan and cook the onion gently for about 5 minutes, until softened. Stir in the crushed garlic and chopped ginger and cook for about 1 minute more.

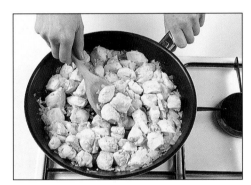

2 Add the chicken cubes to the pan and fry for 2–3 minutes, until they turn white. Crush the cardamom pods and extract the seeds. Add these to the frying pan, with the rest of the spices and the bay leaves. Stir over gentle heat for 1 minute.

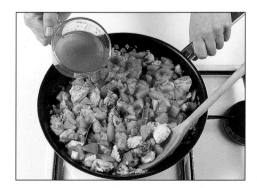

3 Add the lemon juice and chopped tomatoes, then stir in the stock. Bring to a boil, then lower the heat, cover and cook gently for 40 minutes.

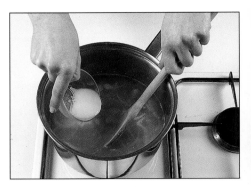

4 Rinse and drain the rice. Warm the milk in a small pan, stir in the saffron and set aside to infuse. Heat the oil in a pan and fry the onion until soft. Stir in the rice, then add the stock and saffron liquid. Bring to a boil, then cover the pan and simmer for about 30 minutes, until the rice is tender and all the stock is absorbed.

5 Layer the rice and chicken in an ovenproof dish, ending with rice. Cover and bake for about 30 minutes, to allow all the flavors to combine.

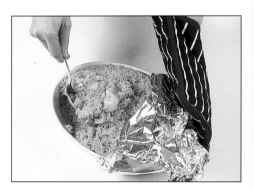

6 Stir gently to bring some of the curry to the top. Sprinkle with rosewater, if using, and garnish with the pistachio nuts, raisins and cilantro. Serve with a bowl of yogurt or raita, if liked.

NUTRITIONAL NOTES
Per Serving

Energy	425 calories
Fat	13.5g
Saturated Fat	3g
Cholesterol	49mg

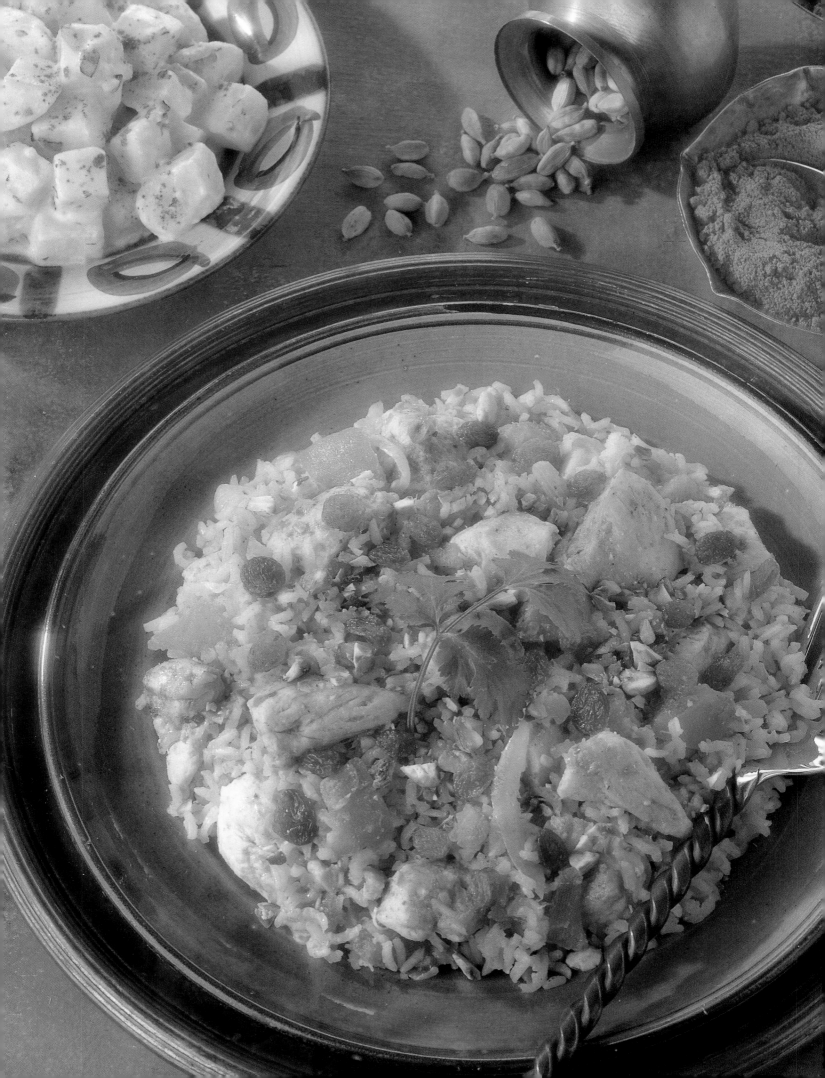

Chicken, Barley and Apple Casserole

Barley supplies valuable minerals and B-group vitamins. This casserole makes a hearty and nourishing cold-weather meal.

INGREDIENTS

Serves 4

4 boneless chicken breasts
1 tablespoon sunflower oil
1 large onion, sliced
1 garlic clove, crushed
3 carrots, cut into chunky sticks
2 celery stalks, thickly sliced
²/₃ cup pot or pearl barley
3 cups chicken stock
1 bay leaf
few sprigs each of fresh thyme and
    marjoram
3 eating apples
chopped fresh parsley, to garnish

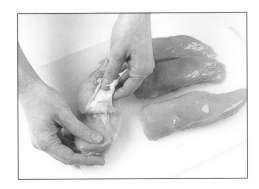

1 Remove the skin from the chicken. Heat the oil and sauté the onion for about 5 minutes until soft.

COOK'S TIP

You can also cook the casserole in a pre-heated 375°F oven. The timings are the same. Chicken thighs are not as "meaty" as chicken breasts, but they are very tasty and less expensive.

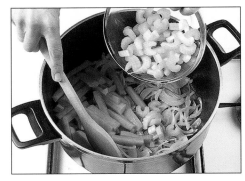

2 Stir in the garlic, carrots and celery and continue to cook over gentle heat for another 5 minutes.

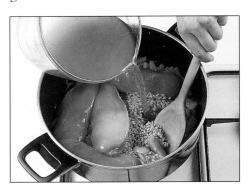

3 Stir in the pearl barley, then add the chicken breasts, stock and herbs. Bring to a boil, then lower the heat, cover the casserole and cook gently for 1 hour.

4 Core the apples and slice them thickly. Add to the casserole, replace the lid and cook for 15 minutes more. Sprinkle with the chopped parsley and serve.

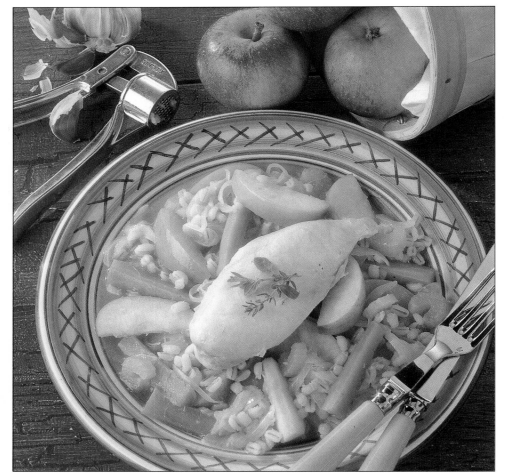

NUTRITIONAL NOTES	
Per Serving	
Energy	355 calories
Fat	9g
Saturated Fat	2g
Cholesterol	64.5mg

Chicken, Banana and Pineapple Kebabs

INGREDIENTS

Serves 4

4 boned chicken thighs, skinned
   and cubed
½ small fresh pineapple
2 firm bananas
fresh orange segments and bay leaves (if
   available), to garnish

For the marinade

3 tablespoons sunflower oil
1 tablespoon clear honey
1 teaspoon French whole-grain mustard
1 teaspoons crushed coriander seeds
grated rind and juice of 1 orange
4 cardamom pods

NUTRITIONAL NOTES	
Per Serving	
Energy	275 calories
Fat	14.5g
Saturated Fat	3g
Cholesterol	73mg

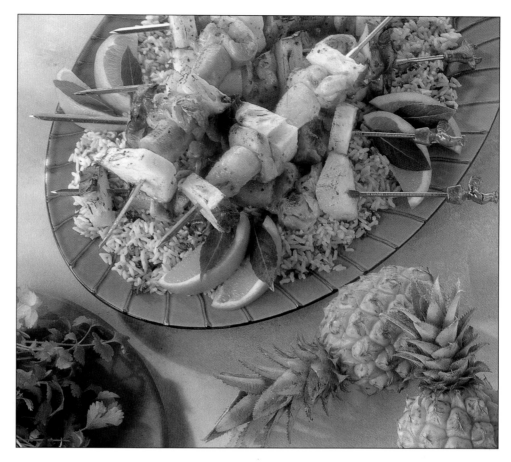

1 Make the marinade. Combine the sunflower oil, clear honey, mustard, coriander seeds and orange rind and juice in a shallow dish. Mix well to combine. Crush the cardamom pods, extract the seeds and stir them into the mixture.

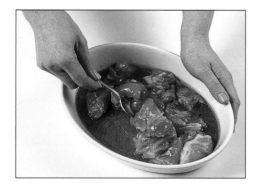

2 Add the prepared chicken cubes to the dish, and turn to coat them all over in the marinade. Then cover the dish and leave to marinate in the fridge for at least 2 hours.

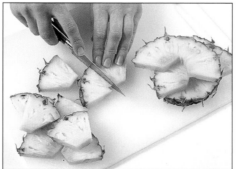

3 Just before cooking, preheat the broiler. Core the pineapple and cut it into neat wedges, leaving the skin on, if you like. Peel and slice the bananas.

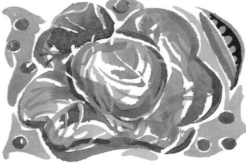

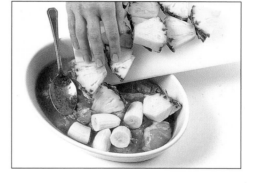

4 Add the pineapple wedges and banana slices to the marinade, coating them thoroughly.

5 Drain the chicken, pineapple and banana, reserving the marinade. Thread alternately on to eight skewers. Broil on a rack under moderate heat, turning the skewers occasionally and brushing them with the reserved marinade, for about 15 minutes until the chicken is golden and cooked through. Garnish with fresh orange segments and bay leaves.

Sweet and Sour Fish

White fish is high in protein, vitamins and minerals, but low in fat. Serve this tasty, nutritious dish with brown rice and stir-fried cabbage or spinach for a delicious lunch-time meal.

INGREDIENTS

Serves 4

4 tablespoons cider vinegar
3 tablespoons light soy sauce
¼ cup granulated sugar
1 tablespoon tomato paste
1½ tablespoons cornstarch
1 cup water
1 green bell pepper, seeded and sliced
8-ounce can pineapple pieces in fruit juice
8 ounces tomatoes, peeled and chopped
2 cups button mushrooms, sliced
1½ pounds chunky haddock fillets, skinned
salt and ground black pepper

1 Preheat the oven to 350°F. Mix the vinegar, soy sauce, sugar and tomato paste in a saucepan. Put the cornstarch in a cup, stir in the water, then add the mixture to the saucepan, stirring well. Bring to a boil, stirring constantly until thickened. Lower the heat and simmer the sauce for 5 minutes.

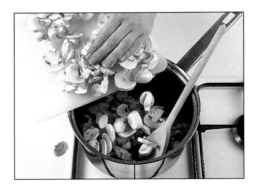

2 Add the green pepper, canned pineapple pieces (with juice), tomatoes and mushrooms to the sauce and heat through. Season to taste with salt and pepper.

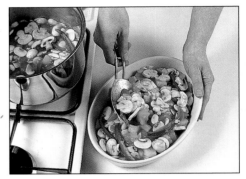

3 Place the fish in a single layer in a shallow ovenproof dish, pour over the sauce and cover with foil. Bake for 15–20 minutes, until the fish is tender. Serve immediately.

NUTRITIONAL NOTES	
Per Serving	
Energy	255 calories
Fat	2g
Saturated Fat	0.5g
Cholesterol	61mg

Tuna and Mixed Vegetable Pasta

INGREDIENTS

Serves 4

2 tablespoons olive oil
1½ cups button mushrooms, sliced
1 garlic clove, crushed
½ red bell pepper, seeded and chopped
1 tablespoon tomato paste
1¼ cups tomato juice
1 cup frozen peas
1–2 tablespoons drained pickled green peppercorns, crushed
2½ cups whole wheat pasta shapes
7-ounce can tuna chunks in water, drained
6 scallions, diagonally sliced

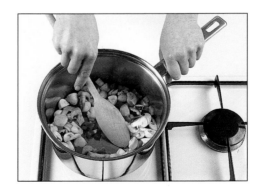

1 Heat the oil in a pan and gently sauté the mushrooms, garlic and pepper until softened. Stir in the tomato paste, then add the tomato juice, peas and some or all of the crushed peppercorns, depending on how spicy you like the sauce. Bring to a boil, lower the heat and simmer.

2 Bring a large saucepan of lightly salted water to a boil and cook the pasta for about 12 minutes (or according to the instructions on the package) until just tender. When the pasta is almost ready, add the tuna to the sauce and heat through gently. Stir in the scallions. Drain the pasta, turn it into a heated bowl, and pour over the sauce. Toss to mix. Serve at once.

NUTRITIONAL NOTES	
Per Serving	
Energy	360 calories
Fat	8g
Saturated Fat	1.5g
Cholesterol	19.5mg

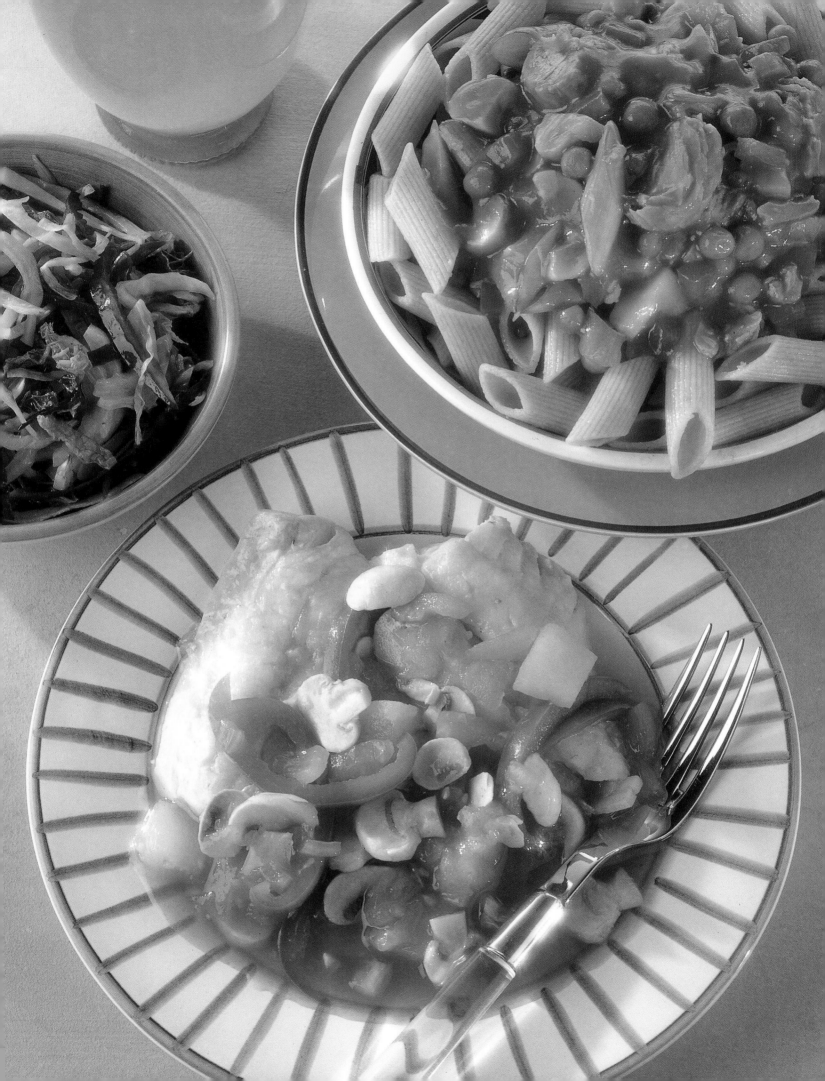

Baked Stuffed Sardines

Oily fish are a good source of vitamins A and D. Serve this nutritious dish with a fresh tomato salad and fresh bread.

INGREDIENTS

Serves 4

12 fresh sardines, scaled and heads removed
1 tablespoon sunflower oil, plus extra for greasing
1 onion, finely chopped
1 garlic clove, crushed
1½ cups fresh whole wheat bread crumbs
1 tablespoon whole-grain mustard
2 tablespoons chopped fresh parsley
1 egg yolk
2 tablespoons grated Parmesan cheese
grated rind and juice of 2 lemons
salt and ground black pepper
lemon and parsley, to garnish

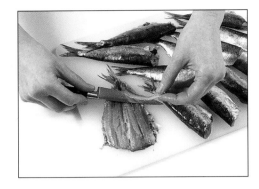

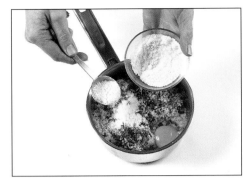

1 Preheat the oven to 375°F. Using a sharp knife, slit the sardines open along their underside, then turn each fish over and press them firmly along the back to loosen the backbone. Remove the backbones and clean and dry the inside of each sardine thoroughly.

2 Heat the oil in a saucepan and sauté the onion and garlic gently until softened and beginning to brown.

3 Remove the pan from the heat and mix in the bread crumbs, mustard, chopped parsley, egg yolk and Parmesan. Stir in half the lemon rind and juice and season to taste.

4 Use the stuffing to fill the cavities of the sardines.

5 Brush a shallow ovenproof dish lightly with oil and add the sardines, in a single layer. Pour over the remaining lemon rind and juice, cover with foil and bake for 30 minutes. Garnish with the lemon wedges and fresh parsley sprigs.

COOK'S TIP

Fresh or frozen sardines are sometimes found in East Coast fish markets where there are large Mediterranean communities. Otherwise, larger oily fish, such as mackerel, herring, or trout could be substituted. Allow one per person.

NUTRITIONAL NOTES
Per Serving

Energy	420 calories
Fat	19g
Saturated Fat	5g
Cholesterol	295mg

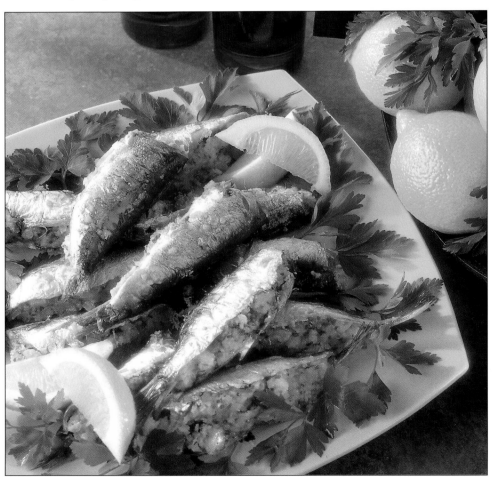

Monkfish with Asparagus and Pears

Monkfish is a superb firm-fleshed fish with a flavor that's often likened to lobster meat. Serve with new potatoes and broccoli.

INGREDIENTS

Serves 4

1 tablespoon sunflower oil
pat of butter, for flavoring (optional)
1 medium onion, sliced
1 garlic clove, crushed
2 zucchini, diagonally sliced
2 firm eating pears, cored
    and sliced
1½ pound monkfish tail, skinned,
    boned and cut into chunks
¾ cup medium-dry white wine
    or cider
¾ cup fish stock
8 ounces asparagus spears, trimmed
strip of pared lemon rind
few fresh dill sprigs
3 tablespoons fat-free sour cream
2 teaspoons cornstarch
salt and ground black pepper
dill sprigs, to garnish

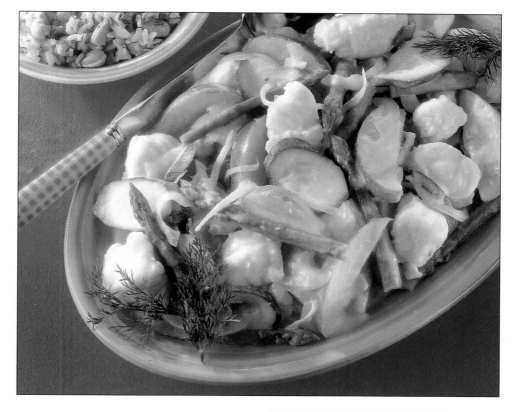

1 Heat the oil (and butter if using) in a large frying pan. Cook the onion, garlic, zucchini and pears over gentle heat for about 5 minutes, until the onion is just beginning to brown. Using a slotted spoon, transfer the mixture to a plate.

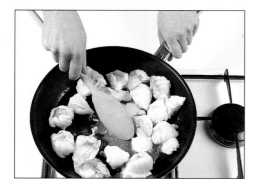

2 Add the monkfish chunks to the fat remaining in the pan and cook for 2–3 minutes, turning frequently, until lightly browned on both sides.

3 Pour in the wine or cider and fish stock and return the vegetables and fruit to the pan.

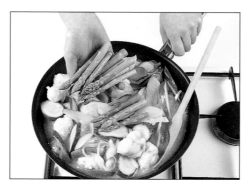

4 Add the asparagus and lemon rind. Season with salt and pepper. Bring to a boil, then lower the heat, cover the pan and simmer gently for about 8 minutes.

5 Add the dill, replace the lid and simmer for 4–7 minutes more, until both the fish and the asparagus are tender. Discard the dill and, using a slotted spoon, remove the fish, fruit and vegetables to a warmed serving dish and keep hot.

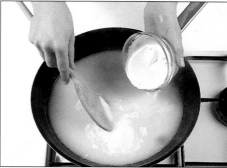

6 Mix the sour cream with the cornstarch in a small bowl, then stir the mixture into the juices remaining in the pan. Cook over gentle heat, stirring constantly, until thickened. Then pour the sauce over the fish and garnish the dish with the dill sprigs.

NUTRITIONAL NOTES	
Per Serving	
Energy	290 calories
Fat	10.5g
Saturated Fat	4g
Cholesterol	55mg

Ginger and Lime Shrimp

INGREDIENTS

Serves 4

8 ounces peeled raw large shrimp
⅓ cucumber
1 tablespoon sunflower oil
1 tablespoon sesame seed oil
6 ounces snow peas, trimmed
4 scallions, diagonally sliced
2 tablespoons chopped cilantro,
  to garnish

For the marinade

1 tablespoon clear honey
1 tablespoon light soy sauce
1 tablespoon dry sherry
2 garlic cloves, crushed
small piece of fresh ginger, peeled and
  finely chopped
juice of 1 lime

1 Mix together the marinade ingredients, add the shrimp and leave to marinate for 1–2 hours.

2 Prepare the cucumber. Slice it in half lengthwise, scoop out the seeds, then slice each half neatly into crescents. Set aside.

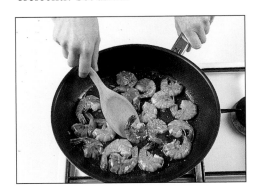

3 Heat both oils in a large heavy-bottomed frying pan or wok. Drain the shrimp (reserving the marinade) and stir-fry over high heat for 4 minutes, until they begin to turn pink. Add the snow peas and the cucumber and stir-fry for 2 minutes more.

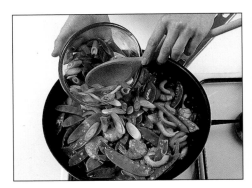

4 Stir in the reserved marinade, heat through, then stir in the scallions and sprinkle with fresh cilantro.

NUTRITIONAL NOTES	
Per Serving	
Energy	140 calories
Fat	6.5g
Saturated Fat	1g
Cholesterol	85mg

Mediterranean Fish Steaks

INGREDIENTS

Serves 4

4 white fish steaks, about 5 ounces
  each
⅔ cup fish stock and/or dry white
  wine, for poaching
1 bay leaf, a few black peppercorns,
  and a strip of pared lemon rind,
  for flavoring
chopped fresh parsley, to garnish

For the tomato sauce

14-ounce can chopped tomatoes
1 garlic clove, crushed
1 tablespoon sun-dried tomato paste
1 tablespoon pastis or other anise-
  flavored liqueur
1 tablespoon drained capers
12–16 pitted black olives
salt and ground black pepper

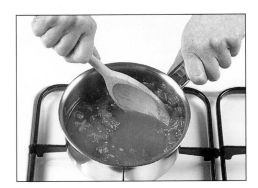

1 Heat together all the tomato sauce ingredients in a pan.

NUTRITIONAL NOTES	
Per Serving	
Energy	165 calories
Fat	3.5g
Saturated Fat	0.5g
Cholesterol	69mg

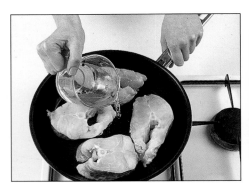

2 Place the fish in a frying pan, pour over the stock and/or wine and add the flavorings. Cover and simmer for 10 minutes, or until it flakes easily.

3 Using a slotted spoon, transfer the fish to a heated dish. Strain the stock into the tomato sauce and boil to reduce slightly. Season the sauce, pour it over the fish and serve immediately, sprinkled with chopped parsley.

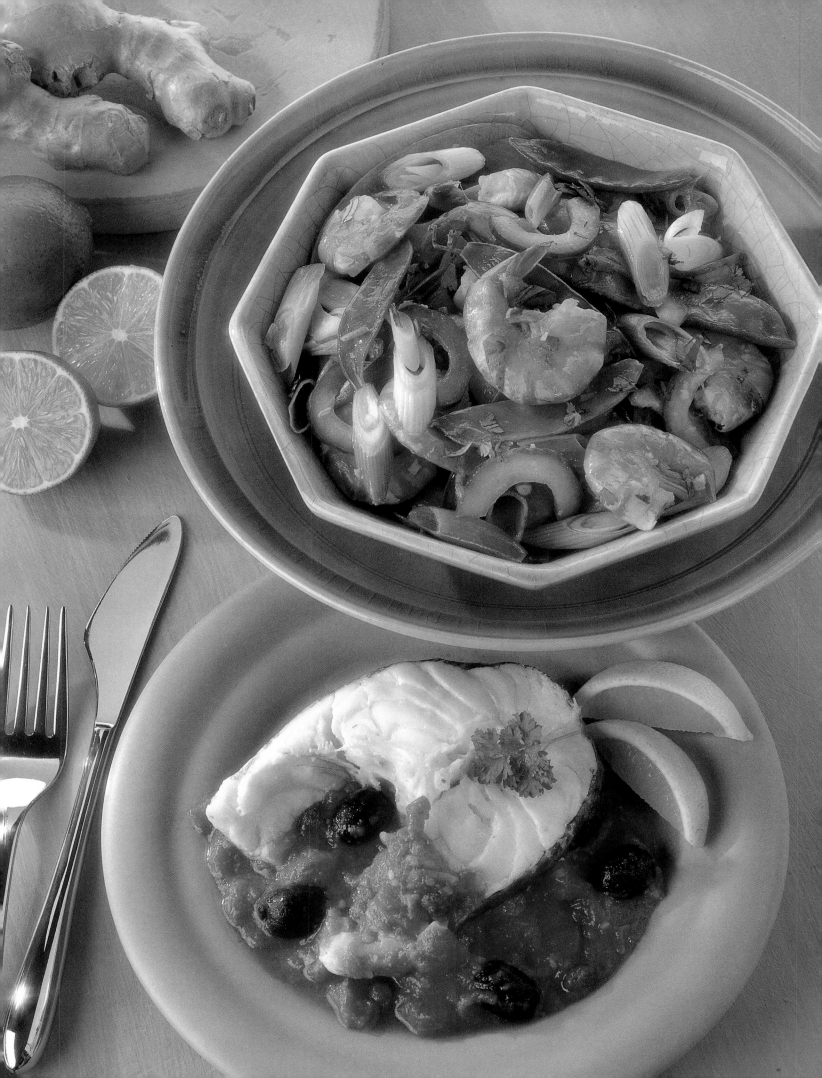

Middle Eastern Rice with Lentils

INGREDIENTS

Serves 4

2 tablespoons sunflower oil
1 large onion, sliced
4 – 5 cardamom pods
½ teaspoon coriander seeds, crushed
½ teaspoon cumin seeds, crushed
small piece of fresh ginger, peeled and
  finely chopped
1 cinnamon stick
1 garlic clove, crushed
⅔ cup brown rice
3¾ cups vegetable stock
½ teaspoon ground turmeric
⅔ cup red lentils
¼ cup flaked almonds, toasted
⅓ cup raisins
low-fat plain yogurt, to serve

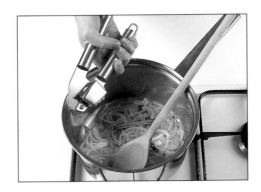

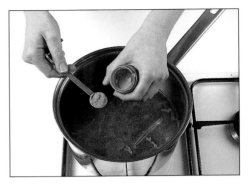

1 Heat the oil in a large saucepan and cook the onion over gentle heat until softened. Crush the cardamom pods, extract the seeds and add them to the pan with the coriander seeds, cumin seeds, ginger, cinnamon stick and garlic. Stir over moderate heat for 2 – 3 minutes.

2 Add the rice, stirring to coat the grains in the spice mixture, then pour in the stock. Stir in the turmeric. Bring to a boil, then lower the heat, cover the pan with a tight-fitting lid and simmer for 15 minutes.

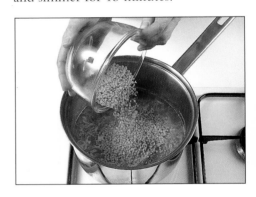

3 Add the lentils to the pan, replace the lid and cook for 20 minutes more, or until the rice and lentils are tender and all the stock has been absorbed (stir in a little more stock if necessary).

4 When all the stock has been absorbed, turn the rice mixture into a heated serving dish and sprinkle the toasted almonds and raisins over the top. Serve with low-fat plain yogurt, if liked.

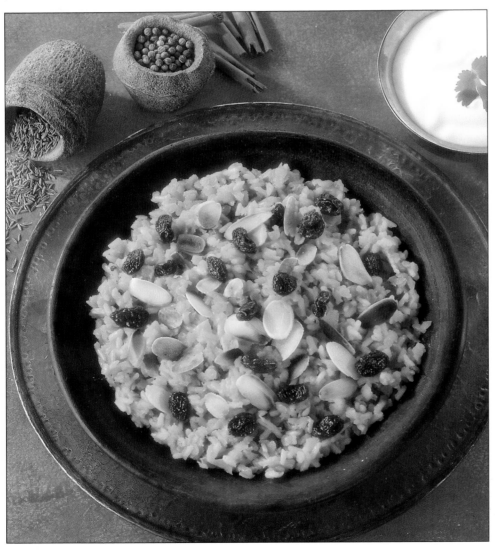

NUTRITIONAL NOTES	
Per Serving	
Energy	350 calories
Fat	11g
Saturated Fat	1.5g
Cholesterol	0

Tagliatelle with Tomato and Zucchini Sauce

INGREDIENTS

Serves 3–4

5–6 ripe tomatoes
8 ounces whole wheat tagliatelle
2 tablespoons olive oil
1 onion, chopped
2 celery stalks, chopped
1 garlic clove, crushed
2 zucchini, sliced
2 tablespoons sun-dried tomato paste
½ cup flaked almonds, toasted
salt and ground black pepper

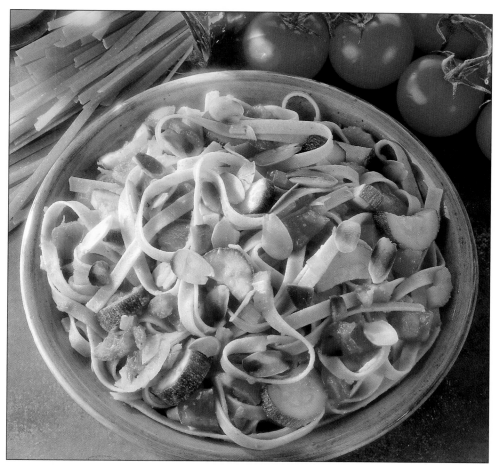

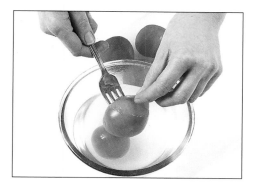

1 Place the tomatoes in a bowl of boiling water for 30 seconds to loosen the skins. Peel, then chop.

2 Bring a large saucepan of lightly salted water to a boil, add the pasta and cook for about 12 minutes (or according to the instructions on the package) until just tender.

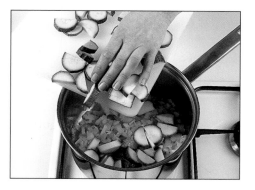

3 Meanwhile, heat the oil in another pan and add the chopped onion, celery, garlic and zucchini. Sauté over gentle heat for 3–4 minutes, or until the onions are softened and become lightly browned.

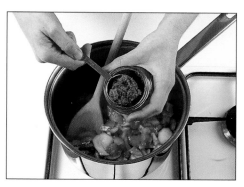

4 Stir in the tomatoes and sun-dried tomato paste. Cook gently for 5 minutes more, then add salt and pepper to taste.

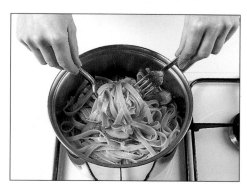

5 Drain the pasta, return it to the pan and add the sauce. Toss well. Place in a serving dish and sprinkle the toasted almonds over the top to serve.

--- COOK'S TIP ---

If using fresh pasta, you'll need to double the quantity, i.e. 1 pound for 3–4 hearty appetites. Fresh tagliatelle usually only takes 3–4 minutes to cook and is ready when it is tender but still *al dente*.

NUTRITIONAL NOTES
Per Serving for 3

Energy	495 calories
Fat	22g
Saturated Fat	2.5g
Cholesterol	0

Chow Mein with Cashew Nuts

INGREDIENTS

Serves 4

2 tablespoons stir-fry oil
½ cup cashew nuts
2 carrots, cut into julienne sticks
3 celery stalks, cut into julienne sticks
1 green bell pepper, seeded and cut
   into thin strips
8 ounces bean sprouts
8 ounces Chinese dried egg noodles
2 tablespoons toasted sesame seeds,
   to garnish

For the lemon sauce

2 tablespoons light soy sauce
1 tablespoon dry sherry
²/₃ cup vegetable stock
2 lemons
1 tablespoon sugar
2 teaspoons cornstarch

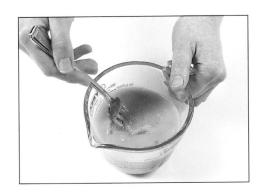

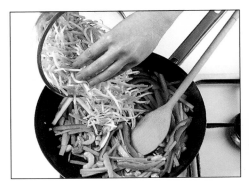

1 Stir all the ingredients for the lemon sauce together in a measuring cup. Bring a large saucepan of lightly salted water to a boil.

2 Heat the oil in a wok or large heavy-bottomed frying pan. Add the cashew nuts, toss quickly over high heat until golden, then remove with a slotted spoon.

3 Add the carrots and celery to the pan and stir-fry for 4–5 minutes. Add the pepper and bean sprouts and stir-fry for 2–3 minutes more.

4 At the same time, cook the noodles in the pan of boiling water for 3 minutes (or according to the instructions on the package).

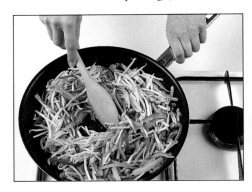

5 Remove the vegetables from the pan with a slotted spoon. Pour in the sauce and cook for 2 minutes, stirring until thick. Return the vegetables to the pan, add the cashew nuts and stir quickly to coat in sauce.

6 Drain the noodles when cooked, turn them into a serving dish and spoon the vegetables and sauce over. Sprinkle with sesame seeds and serve.

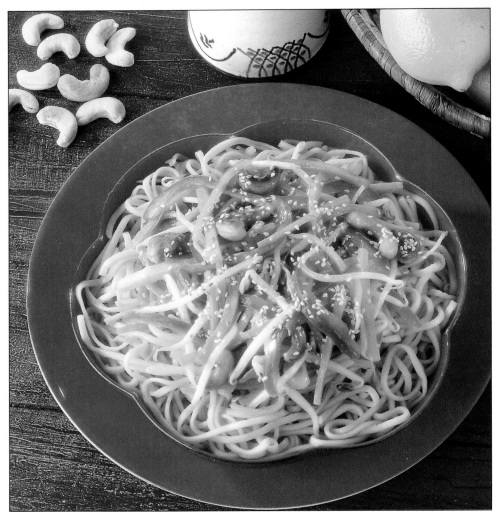

NUTRITIONAL NOTES	
Per Serving	
Energy	460 calories
Fat	21.5g
Saturated Fat	2.5g
Cholesterol	25mg

Mushroom and Mixed Nut Roast

INGREDIENTS

Serves 4

3 tablespoons sunflower seeds
3 tablespoons sesame seeds
2 tablespoons sunflower oil, plus extra
  for greasing
1 onion, coarsely chopped
2 celery stalks, coarsely chopped
1 green bell pepper, seeded and
  chopped
2 cups mixed wild and cultivated
  mushrooms, chopped
1 garlic clove, crushed
2 cups fresh whole wheat bread crumbs
1 cup chopped mixed nuts
⅓ cup golden raisins
small piece of fresh ginger, peeled and
  finely chopped
2 teaspoons coriander seeds, crushed
2 tablespoons light soy sauce
1 egg, beaten
salt and ground black pepper
celery and cilantro leaves, to garnish

For the tomato sauce

14-ounce can chopped tomatoes
3 scallions, chopped
2 tablespoons chopped cilantro

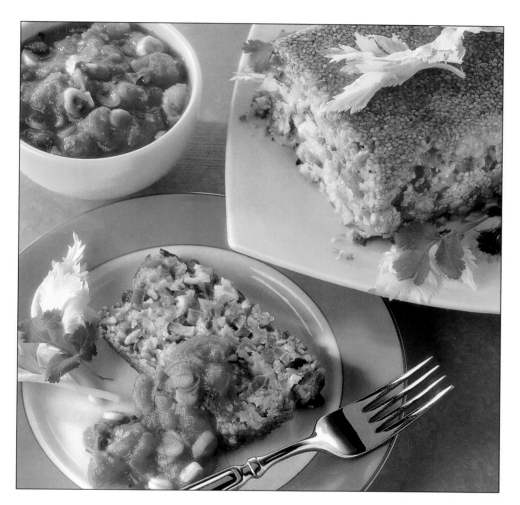

NUTRITIONAL NOTES	
Per Serving	
Energy	460 calories
Fat	37.5g
Saturated Fat	4.5g
Cholesterol	53mg

2 Preheat the oven to 375°F. Heat
the oil in a frying pan, add the
onion, celery, pepper, mushrooms and
garlic and cook over gentle heat for
about 5 minutes, until the onion has
softened.

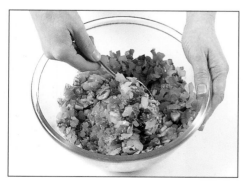

3 Mix the bread crumbs and nuts in
a large bowl. Add the contents of
the frying pan, then stir in the raisins,
ginger, coriander seeds and soy sauce.
Mix with the egg, then season.

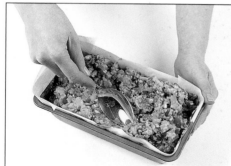

4 Press the mixture evenly into the
pan and bake for 45 minutes.
Make the sauce. Heat the tomatoes in a
small saucepan, add the scallions and
cilantro and season to taste.

5 When the loaf is cooked, loosen it
with a knife, then allow to cool
for a few minutes. Turn out onto a
serving dish and garnish with the celery
and cilantro leaves. Serve with the
warm tomato sauce.

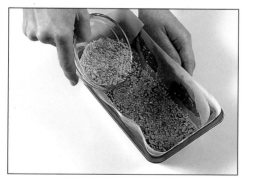

1 Grease and line a 1½-pound loaf
pan. Sprinkle the sunflower and
sesame seeds on the bottom.

Spicy Bean Hotpot

INGREDIENTS

Serves 4

2 cups mushrooms
1 tablespoon sunflower oil
2 onions, sliced
1 garlic clove, crushed
1 tablespoon red wine vinegar
14-ounce can chopped tomatoes
1 tablespoon tomato paste
1 tablespoon Worcestershire sauce or
  brown sauce
1 tablespoon whole-grain mustard
1 tablespoon dark brown sugar
1 cup vegetable stock
14-ounce can red kidney
  beans, drained
14-ounce can navy or cannellini
  beans, drained
1 bay leaf
½ cup raisins
salt and ground black pepper
chopped fresh parsley, to garnish

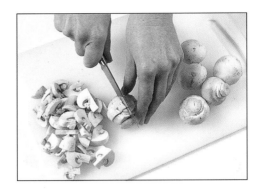

1 Wipe the mushrooms, then use a sharp vegetable knife to cut them into small pieces and set aside.

2 Heat the oil in a large saucepan or flameproof casserole, add the onions and garlic and cook over gentle heat for 10 minutes until soft.

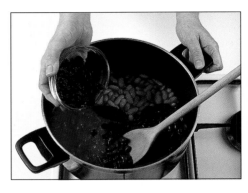

3 Add all the remaining ingredients except the mushrooms and seasoning. Bring to a boil, lower the heat, and simmer for 10 minutes.

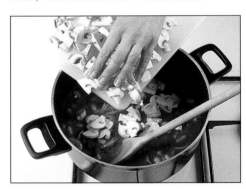

4 Add the mushrooms and simmer for 5 minutes more. Stir in salt and pepper to taste. Transfer to a heated serving dish and sprinkle with parsley.

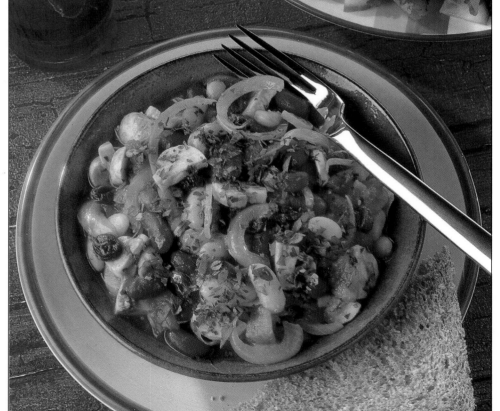

NUTRITIONAL NOTES	
Per Serving	
Energy	280 calories
Fat	4.5g
Saturated Fat	0.5g
Cholesterol	0

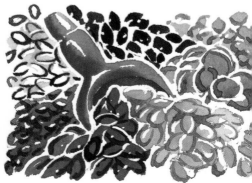

Chick-pea and Spinach Curry

Chick-peas provide protein, minerals and B-group vitamins to this tasty low-fat, high-fiber curry, while spinach is a valuable vegetable source of iron. Serve this curry with brown rice or nan bread and a yogurt raita or chutney, if you like.

INGREDIENTS

Serves 3–4

2 tablespoons sunflower oil
1 large onion, finely chopped
2 garlic cloves, crushed
1-inch piece of fresh ginger, peeled and
    finely chopped
1 green chili, seeded and finely
    chopped
2 tablespoons medium curry paste
2 teaspoons ground cumin
1 teaspoon ground turmeric
8-ounce can chopped tomatoes
1 green or red bell pepper, seeded
    and chopped
1¼ cups vegetable stock
1 tablespoon tomato paste
1 pound fresh spinach
15-ounce can chick-peas, drained
3 tablespoons chopped cilantro
salt
1 teaspoon garam masala (optional)

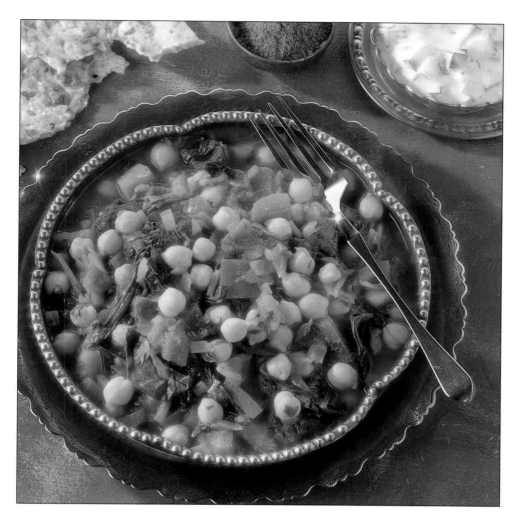

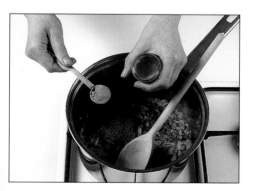

1 Heat the sunflower oil in a large saucepan or flameproof casserole. Then add the chopped onion, crushed garlic, fresh ginger and green chili. Cook over gentle heat for about 5 minutes, or until the onions are softened but not browned.

2 Stir in the curry paste, cook for 1 minute more, then stir in the cumin and turmeric. Continue stirring over low heat for 1 minute more.

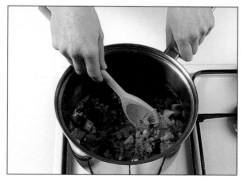

3 Add the tomatoes and pepper to the pan and stir to coat with the spice mixture. Pour in the stock and stir in the tomato paste. Bring to a boil, lower the heat, cover and simmer for 15 minutes.

4 Remove any coarse stalks from the spinach, chop the leaves coarsely and add them to the pan. You will probably have to do this in batches, as fresh spinach leaves are rather bulky. They cook down after about 1 minute, so this will not take very long.

5 Add the chick-peas, cover and cook gently for 5 minutes more. Stir in the cilantro, season with salt and sprinkle with garam masala, if using. Serve at once.

NUTRITIONAL NOTES	
Per Serving for 3	
Energy	315 calories
Fat	15g
Saturated Fat	1.5g
Cholesterol	0

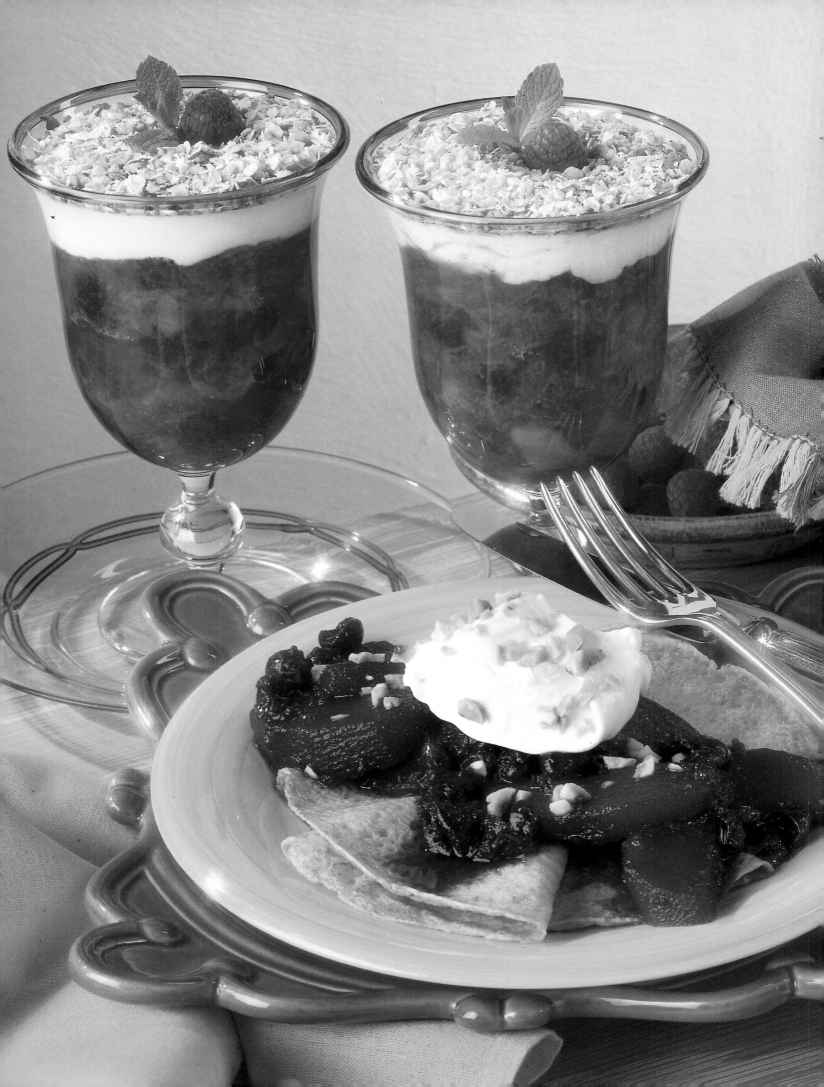

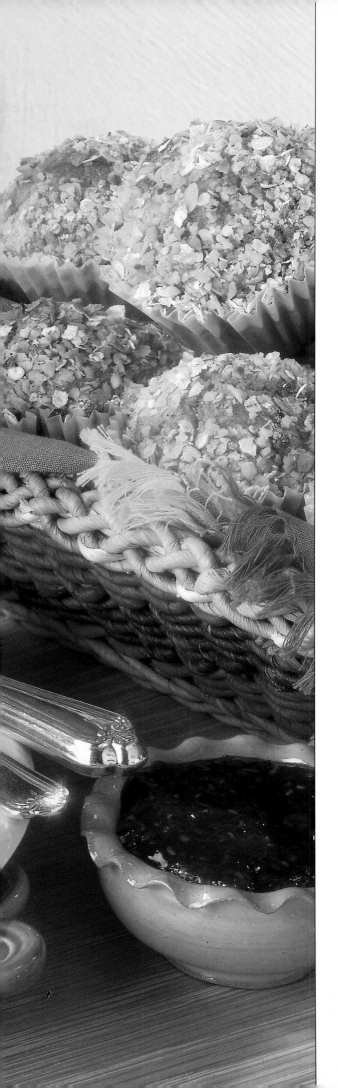

Desserts and Sweet Breads

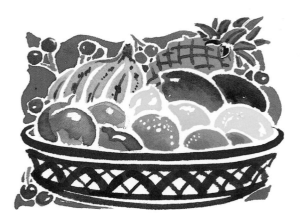

This is where, so often, good intentions give way to weakness and temptation. Most sweets and creamy desserts are loaded with fat and sugar and are low on nutritional value – they won't help you on the road to fitness and vitality. However, there's still a place for sweet treats made with whole-grain cereals, fruits, nuts and low-fat substitutes for the richer dairy products. This mouthwatering selection shows how easily sweet recipes may be adapted to healthier versions.

Autumn Pudding

Summer pudding is far too good to be reserved for the summer berry season. Here is an autumn version, with apples, plums and blackberries, which makes a high-fiber dessert full of vitamins.

INGREDIENTS

Serves 6
1 pound eating apples
1 pound plums, halved and pitted
8 ounces blackberries, hulled
4 tablespoons apple juice
sugar or honey, to sweeten (optional)
8 slices of whole wheat bread,
   crusts removed
mint sprig and blackberry, to decorate
fat-free sour cream, to serve

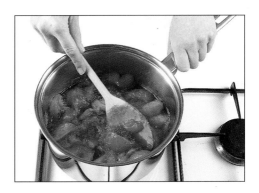

1 Quarter the apples, remove the cores and peel, then slice them into a saucepan. Add the plums, blackberries and apple juice. Cover and cook gently for 10 – 15 minutes or until tender. Sweeten, if necessary, with a little sugar or honey, although the fruit should be sweet enough.

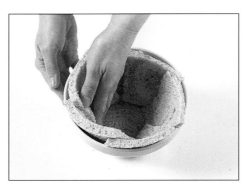

2 Line the bottom and sides of a 5 cup pudding mold with 6 – 7 slices of bread, cut to fit. Press together tightly.

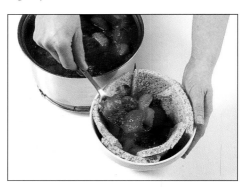

3 Spoon the fruit into the mold. Pour in just enough juice to moisten. Reserve any remaining juice.

4 Cover the fruit completely with the remaining bread. Fit a plate on top, so that it rests on the bread just below the rim. Stand the mold in a larger bowl to catch any juice. Place a weight on the plate and chill overnight.

5 Turn the pudding out on to a plate and pour the reserved juice over any areas which have not absorbed the juice. Decorate with the mint sprig and blackberry and serve with sour cream.

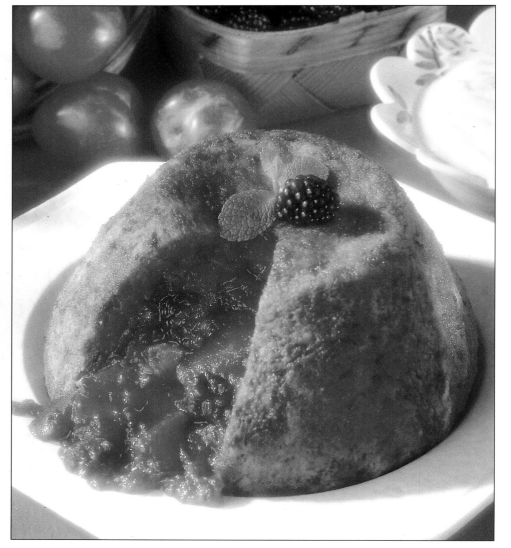

NUTRITIONAL NOTES	
Per Serving	
Energy	185 calories
Fat	1.5g
Saturated Fat	0.5g
Cholesterol	0

Fragrant Rice with Mango Purée

Nuts, dried fruit, cardamom and rosewater make this Indian-style rice pudding a real treat.

INGREDIENTS

Serves 6

2 ripe mangoes
⅓ cup basmati rice
6 cups low-fat milk
⅓ cup raw sugar
⅓ cup golden raisins
1 teaspoon rosewater
5 cardamom pods
3 tablespoons orange juice
scant ¼ cup flaked
  almonds, toasted
scant ¼ cup pistachio
  nuts, chopped

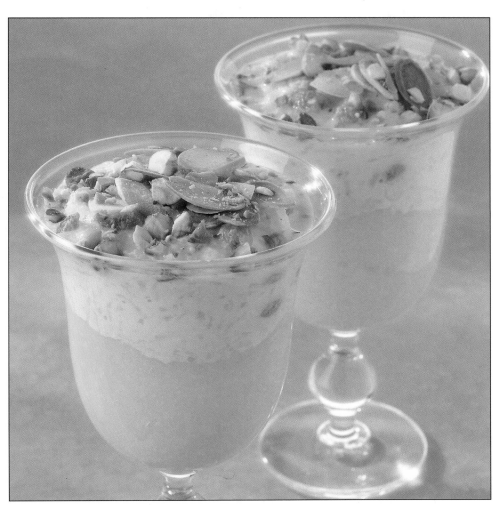

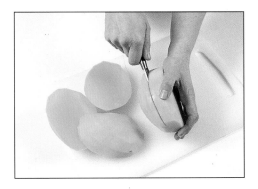

1 Using a sharp knife, peel, slice and pit the mangoes.

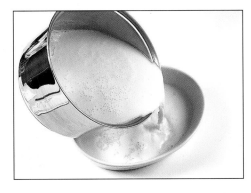

2 Preheat the oven to 300°F. Put the basmati rice in an ovenproof dish. Boil the milk then pour it over the rice. Bake uncovered for 2 hours, until the rice has become soft and mushy.

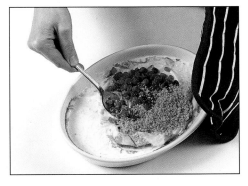

3 Remove the dish from the oven and stir in the raw sugar and raisins, with half the rosewater. Crush the cardamom pods, extract the seeds and stir them into the rice mixture. Allow to cool.

4 Place the mango flesh in a blender or food processor. Add the orange juice and remaining rosewater. Blend until smooth.

5 Divide the mango purée among six individual glass serving dishes. Spoon the rice pudding mixture evenly over the top. Leave to chill thoroughly in the fridge or a cool place.

6 When ready to serve, sprinkle the toasted almonds and chopped pistachio nuts over the top of each dessert.

NUTRITIONAL NOTES	
Per Serving	
Energy	300 calories
Fat	8g
Saturated Fat	3g
Cholesterol	17.5mg

Fruit Fondue with Hazelnut Dip

INGREDIENTS

Serves 2

selection of fresh fruits for dipping,
  such as clementines, kiwi fruit,
  grapes, physalis and whole
  strawberries
½ cup low-fat soft cheese
⅔ cup low-fat plain yogurt
¼ cup chopped hazelnuts
1 teaspoon vanilla extract
1 teaspoon superfine sugar

NUTRITIONAL NOTES *Per Serving (Dip only)*	
Energy	170 calories
Fat	4g
Saturated Fat	2.5g
Cholesterol	6.5mg

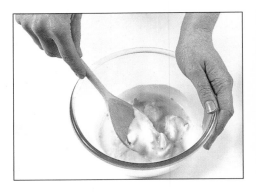

1 First prepare the fruits. Peel and segment the clementines. Then peel the kiwi fruit and cut into wedges. Wash the grapes and peel back the papery casing on the physalis.

2 Beat the soft cheese with the yogurt, vanilla extract and sugar in a bowl. Stir in three-quarters of the hazelnuts. Spoon the dip into a glass serving dish set on a platter or small pots on individual plates and scatter over the remaining hazelnuts. Arrange the prepared fruits around the dip and serve immediately.

Yogurt Sundaes with Passionfruit Coulis

Here is a sundae you can enjoy every day! The frozen yogurt has less fat and fewer calories than traditional ice cream and the fruits provide vitamins A and C.

INGREDIENTS

Serves 4

12 ounces strawberries, halved
2 passionfruits, halved
2 teaspoons confectioner's sugar
  (optional)
2 ripe peaches, pitted and chopped
8 scoops (about 12 ounces) vanilla or
  strawberry frozen yogurt

NUTRITIONAL NOTES *Per Serving*	
Energy	135 calories
Fat	1g
Saturated Fat	0.5g
Cholesterol	3.5mg

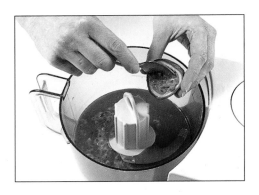

1 Purée half the strawberries. Scoop out the passionfruit pulp and add it to the coulis. Sweeten, if necessary.

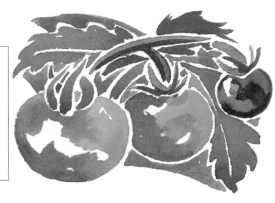

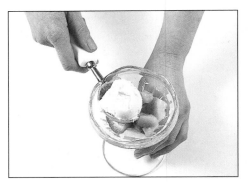

2 Spoon half the remaining strawberries and half the chopped peaches into four tall sundae glasses. Top each dessert with a scoop of frozen yogurt. Set aside a few choice pieces of fruit for decoration, and use the rest to make another layer on the top of each sundae. Top each with a final scoop of frozen yogurt.

3 Pour over the passionfruit coulis and decorate the sundaes with the reserved strawberries and pieces of peach. Serve immediately.

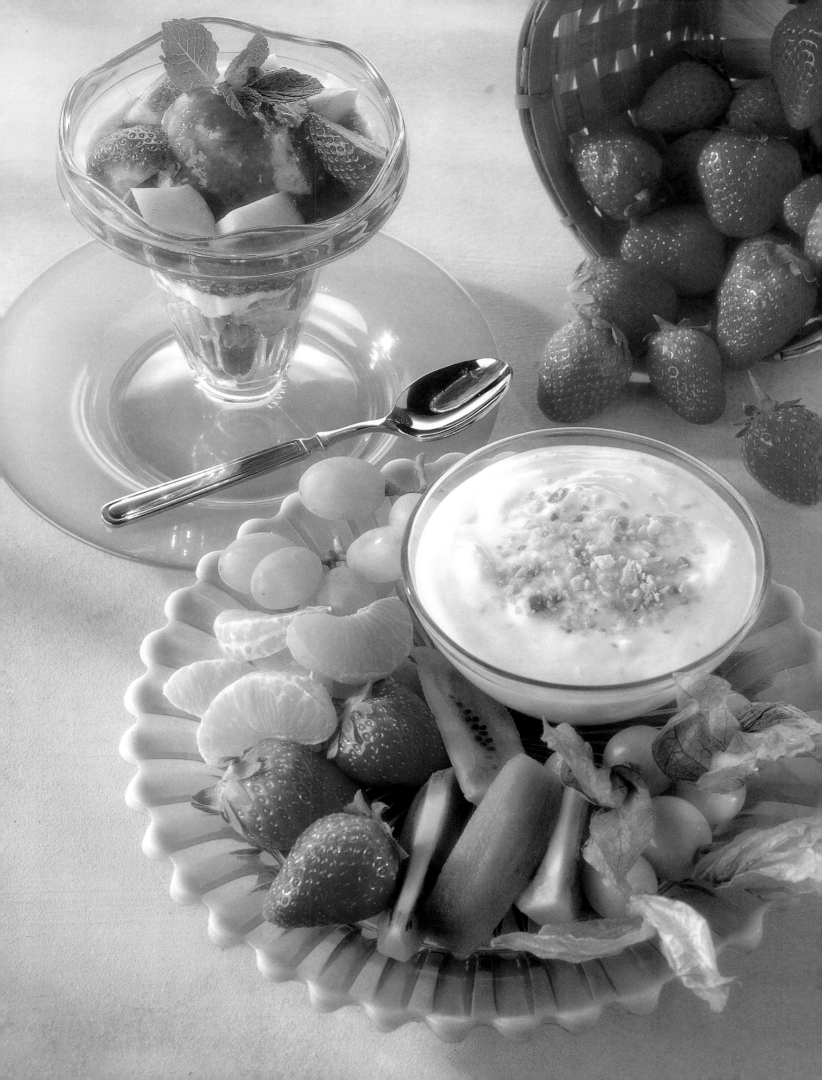

Apple and Black Currant Crêpes

These crêpes are made with a whole wheat batter and are filled with a delicious fruit mixture.

INGREDIENTS

Makes 8–10
1 cup whole wheat flour
1¼ cups skimmed milk
1 egg, beaten
1 tablespoon sunflower oil, plus extra
    for greasing
low-fat plain yogurt, to serve (optional)
toasted nuts or sesame seeds, for
    sprinkling (optional)

For the filling
1 pound cooking apples
8 ounces black currants
2–3 tablespoons water
2 tablespoons raw sugar

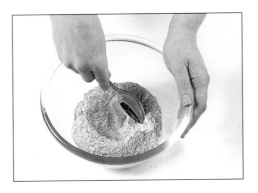

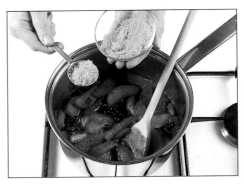

1 Make the crêpe batter. Place the flour in a mixing bowl and make a well in the center.

2 Add a little of the milk with the egg and the oil. Whisk the flour into the liquid, then gradually whisk in the rest of the milk, keeping the batter smooth and free from lumps. Cover the batter and chill while you prepare the filling.

3 Quarter, peel and core the apples. Slice them into a pan and add the black currants and water. Cook over gentle heat for 10–15 minutes or until the fruit is soft. Stir in enough raw sugar to sweeten.

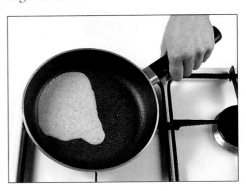

4 Lightly grease a griddle with just a smear of oil. Heat the pan, pour in about 2 tablespoons batter, swirl it around and cook for about 1 minute. Flip the crêpe over with a spatula and cook the other side. Keep hot while cooking the remaining crêpes (unless cooking to order).

5 Fill the crêpes with the apple and black currant mixture and roll them up. Serve with a dollop of yogurt, if using, and sprinkle with nuts or sesame seeds, if desired.

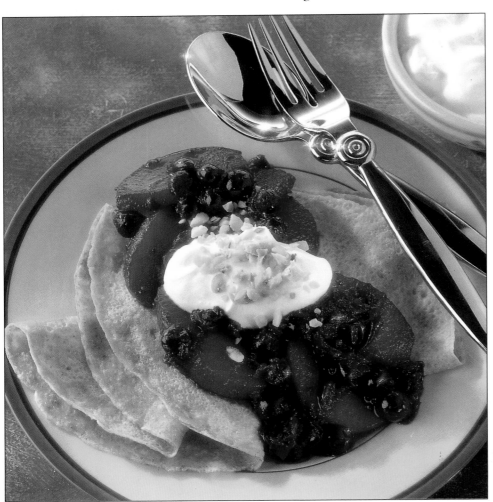

NUTRITIONAL NOTES	
Per Serving for 8	
Energy	120 calories
Fat	3g
Saturated Fat	0.5g
Cholesterol	25mg

Warm Bagels with Poached Apricots

INGREDIENTS

Serves 4

a few strips of orange peel
1⅓ cups dried apricots
1 cup fresh orange juice
½ teaspoon orange flower water
2 cinnamon and raisin bagels
4 teaspoons pure fruit orange
   marmalade
4 tablespoons fat-free sour cream
2 tablespoons chopped pistachio nuts,
   to decorate

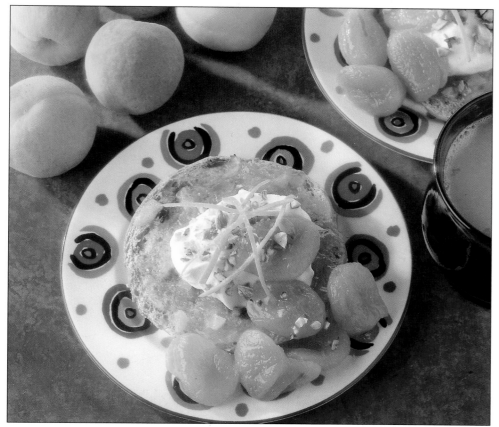

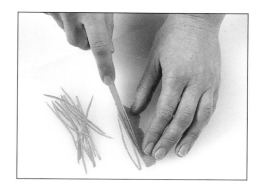

1 Cut the strips of orange peel into fine shreds. Place them in boiling water until softened, then drain and place in cold water.

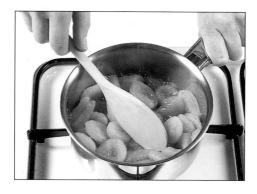

2 Preheat the oven to 325°F. Combine the apricots and orange juice in a small saucepan. Heat gently for about 10 minutes, until the juice has reduced and looks syrupy. Allow to cool, then stir in the orange flower water. Meanwhile, place the bagels on a baking sheet and warm in the oven for 5–10 minutes.

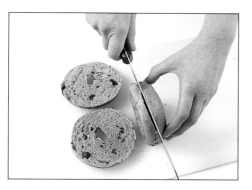

3 Split the bagels in half horizontally. Lay one half, inside uppermost, on each serving plate. Spread 1 teaspoon orange marmalade on each bagel.

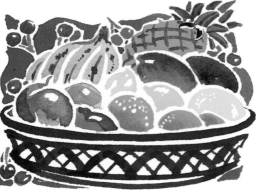

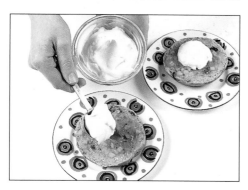

4 Spoon 1 tablespoon fat-free sour cream into the center of each bagel and place a quarter of the apricot compôte at the side. Sprinkle orange peel and pistachio nuts over the top to decorate. Serve immediately.

NUTRITIONAL NOTES	
Per Serving for 8	
Energy	260 calories
Fat	9g
Saturated Fat	4g
Cholesterol	51.5mg

Cranberry Oat Bars

Here's a real tea-time treat for everybody to enjoy!

INGREDIENTS

Makes 14

1½ cups rolled oats
²/₃ cup raw sugar
½ cup dried cranberries
½ cup polyunsaturated margarine,
  melted
oil, for greasing

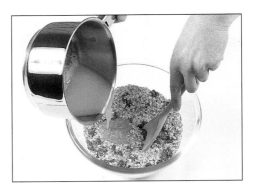

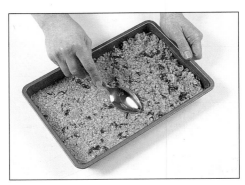

2 Stir the oats, sugar and cranberries together in a bowl. Pour in the melted margarine and stir thoroughly until combined.

3 Press the oat and cranberry mixture into the prepared pan. Bake for 15–20 minutes, until golden.

4 Remove the pan from the oven and score the cake lightly into 14 bars, then leave to cool for 5 minutes, in the pan. Remove the bars and place on a wire rack to cool completely. Store for up to 5 days in an airtight container.

COOK'S TIP

Dried cranberries are a relatively new product, available from larger supermarkets. They have a sweet yet slightly tart flavor and their bright red color will add visual appeal. They can be used to replace more usual dried fruits.

NUTRITIONAL NOTES	
Per Bar	
Energy	150 calories
Fat	8g
Saturated Fat	1.5g
Cholesterol	0.5mg

1 Preheat the oven to 375°F. Grease a shallow 11- x 7-inch pan.

Rhubarb and Raspberry Sundaes

INGREDIENTS

Serves 4

12 ounces rhubarb
2 tablespoons unsweetened
  orange juice
6 ounces raspberries
2 tablespoons pure fruit raspberry jam
⅓ cup rolled oats
¼ cup mixed chopped nuts
scant 1 cup low-fat vanilla yogurt

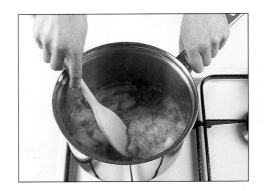

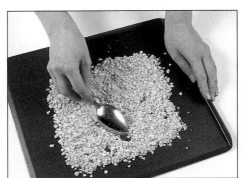

1 Cut the rhubarb into chunks. Heat the orange juice in a saucepan and poach the rhubarb gently for 8–10 minutes, until just tender. Remove from the heat immediately. Allow to cool, then stir in the raspberries and pure fruit jam.

2 Spread the oats and nuts out on a baking sheet and toast them briefly under a hot broiler.

3 Spoon the fruit mixture into four sundae dishes. Top each portion with yogurt, then sprinkle the toasted oats and nuts over the top.

NUTRITIONAL NOTES	
Per Serving	
Energy	135 calories
Fat	5.5g
Saturated Fat	1g
Cholesterol	2mg

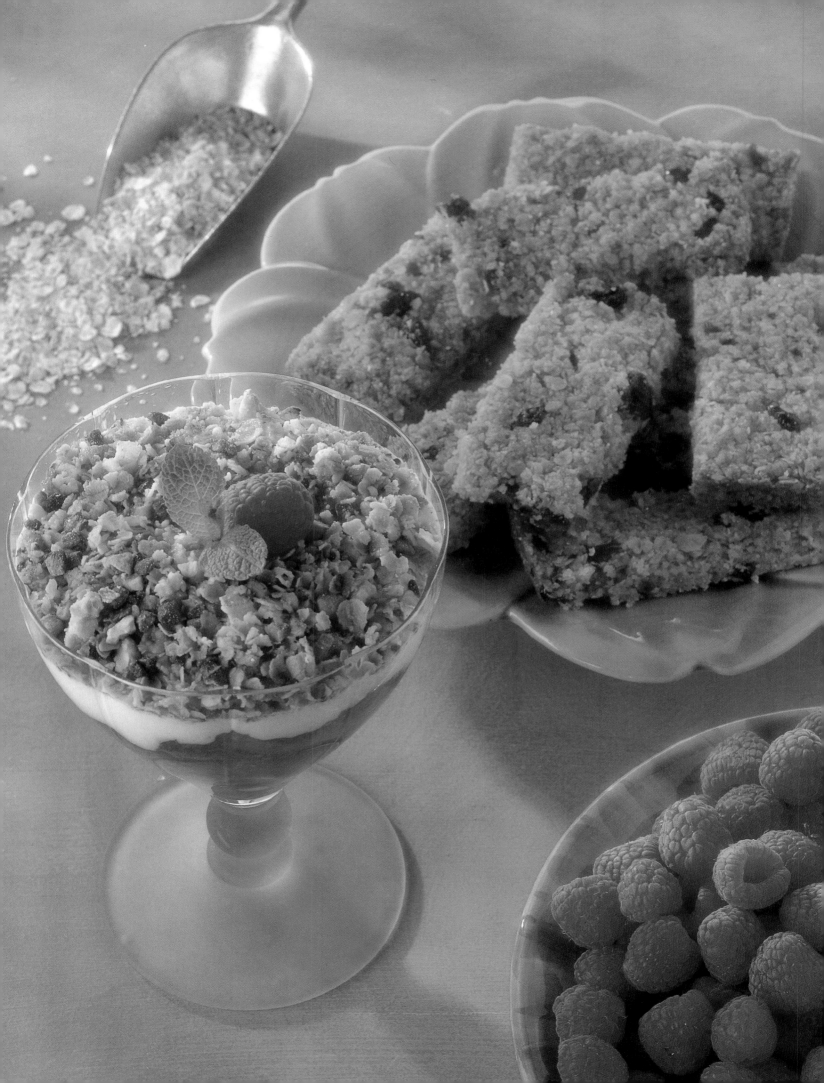

Whole Wheat Apple, Apricot and Walnut Loaf

INGREDIENTS

Makes 10–12 slices
2 cups whole wheat flour
1 teaspoon baking powder
pinch of salt
½ cup sunflower or low-fat margarine
1 cup light brown sugar
2 large eggs, lightly beaten
grated rind and juice of 1 orange
½ cup chopped walnuts
⅓ cup dried apricots, chopped
1 large cooking apple
oil, for greasing

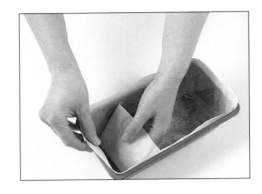

1 Preheat the oven to 350°F. Grease a 2-pound loaf pan and line with wax paper.

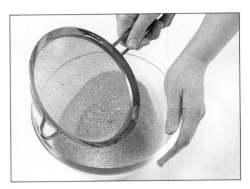

2 Sift the flour, baking powder and salt into a large mixing bowl, then turn the bran remaining in the sieve into the mixture. Add the margarine, sugar, eggs, orange rind and juice. Stir, then beat with a hand-held electric beater until smooth.

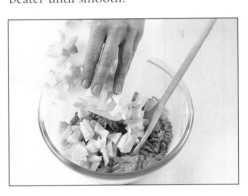

3 Stir in the walnuts and apricots. Quarter, peel and core the apple, chop it coarsely and add it to the mixture. Stir, then spoon the mixture into the prepared pan and level the top.

4 Bake for 1 hour, or until a skewer inserted into the center of the loaf comes out clean. Cool in the pan for about 5 minutes, then turn the loaf out on to a wire rack and peel off the lining paper. When cold, store in an airtight tin.

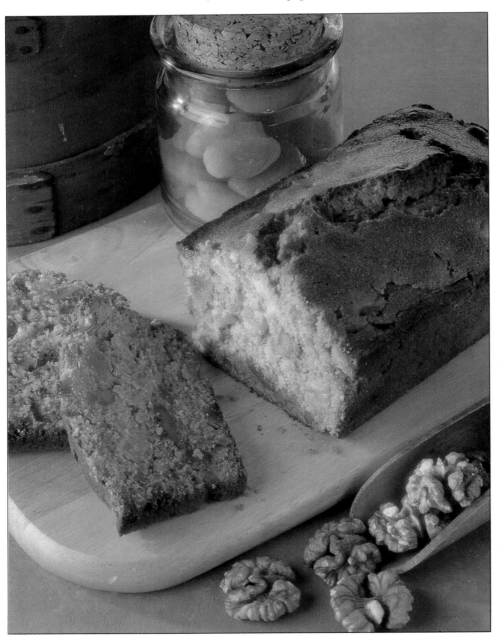

NUTRITIONAL NOTES	
Per Slice if making 10	
Energy	290 calories
Fat	14.5g
Saturated Fat	2.5g
Cholesterol	43.5mg

Spiced Banana Muffins

Whole wheat muffins, with banana for added fiber, make a delicious treat at any time of the day. If preferred, slice off the tops and fill with a teaspoon of reduced-sugar jam or marmalade.

INGREDIENTS

Makes 12

¾ cup whole wheat flour
½ cup all-purpose flour
2 teaspoons baking powder
pinch of salt
1 teaspoon mixed ground cinnamon,
  nutmeg, and allspice
¼ cup light brown sugar
¼ cup polyunsaturated or low-fat
  margarine
1 egg, beaten
⅔ cup low-fat milk
grated rind of 1 orange
1 ripe banana
¼ cup rolled oats
scant ¼ cup chopped hazelnuts

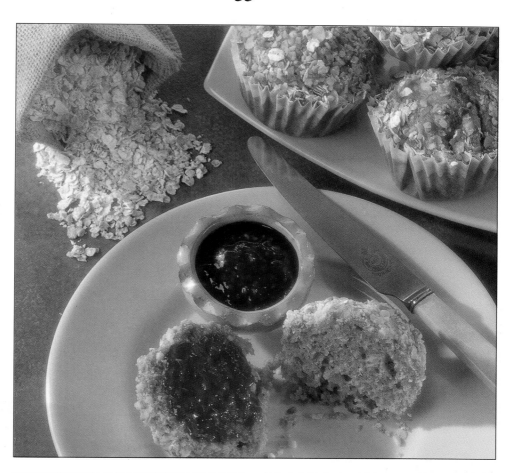

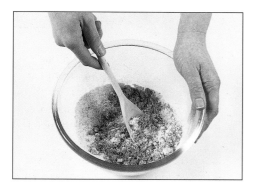

1 Preheat the oven to 400°F. Line a muffin pan with 12 large paper cups. Sift together both flours, the baking powder, salt and mixed spices into a bowl, then turn the bran remaining in the sieve into the bowl. Stir in the sugar.

2 Melt the margarine and pour it into a mixing bowl. Cool slightly, then beat in the egg, milk and grated orange rind.

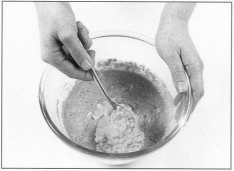

3 Gently fold in the dry ingredients. Mash the banana with a fork, then stir it gently into the mixture, being careful not to overmix.

NUTRITIONAL NOTES	
Per Muffin	
Energy	110 calories
Fat	5g
Saturated Fat	1g
Cholesterol	17.5mg

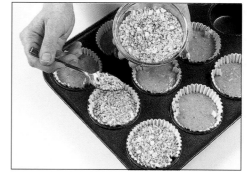

4 Spoon the mixture into the paper cases. Combine the oats and hazelnuts and sprinkle a little of the mixture over each muffin.

5 Bake for 20 minutes, until the muffins are well risen and golden, and a skewer inserted in the center comes out clean. Transfer to a wire rack and serve warm or cold.

Index